CHAKRA
Healing for
CATS

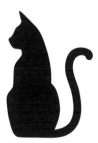

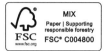

Published in 2022 by OH! Life
An imprint of Welbeck Non-Fiction Limited, part of Welbeck Publishing Group.
Based in London and Sydney.
www.welbeckpublishing.com

Text © Lynn McKenzie 2022
Design © Welbeck Non-Fiction Limited 2022
Illustrations by Sian Summerhayes © Welbeck Non-Fiction Limited 2022

Cover images: Sian Summerhayes © Welbeck Non-Fiction Limited (front);
Shutterstock/Anne Mathiasz and /J.FLA (back), /Mary Erskine (spine).

A CIP catalogue record for this book is available from the British Library.

ISBN 978-1-83861-088-3

Associate Publisher: Lisa Dyer
Copyeditor: Katie Hewett
Designer: Lucy Palmer
Production Controller: Felicity Awdry
Indexer: Vanessa Bird

Printed and bound in Dubai

10 9 8 7 6 5 4 3 2 1

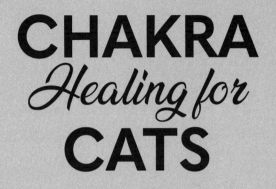

CHAKRA
Healing for
CATS

Energy work for a happy
and healthy feline friend

LYNN MCKENZIE

Illustrations by Sian Summerhayes

CONTENTS

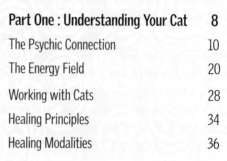

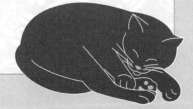

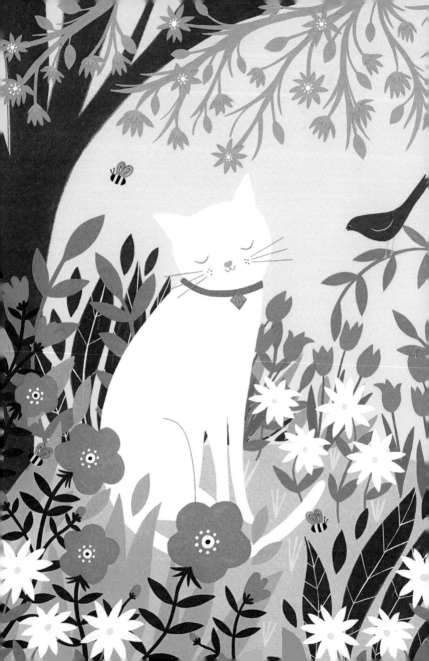

PREFACE

This book was created to teach – and awaken you to – everything you need to know about the chakras of cats. Some of the things you'll learn include what chakras are; where they are located; how you can detect and balance them for greater health and wellbeing for your feline companion; how you can connect more closely with your cat and help them tremendously by working with their chakras; and even how your own chakras are connected to your cat's. Understanding how chakras play a key role in all aspects of your cat's health – physical, emotional, mental and spiritual – is vital to the overall picture of their wellbeing. You will also learn about the energy field as a whole and how it factors into balancing the chakras to heal and benefit your cat.

While the knowledge of chakras and their role is crucial when assessing your cat's health, it's important to always err on the side of safety and common sense when working on your cat's chakras for healing. Consult a veterinarian to rule out illness if you observe any changes in the health or behaviour of your feline friend. Please also note that as you learn more about cats and healing their chakras, when we refer to your cat as "she", we are talking about both female and male cats. Also, the terms "chakra balancing", "chakra clearing" and "chakra healing" are used interchangeably throughout.

There are several approaches to use when balancing your cat's chakras. If your cat has a specific issue she needs help with, you can look up the corresponding chakra(s) and work with it or them, as in Part Two of this book. You can also use the energy methods described in Part One to determine which chakras need balancing and set the intention that working from this perspective will help alleviate any current or future issues. Part Three offers whole-body work using crystals, essences, elixirs and pendulum dowsing. With all this in mind, prepare to embark on a healing journey that may very well provide positive and memorable experiences for both you and your feline friend.

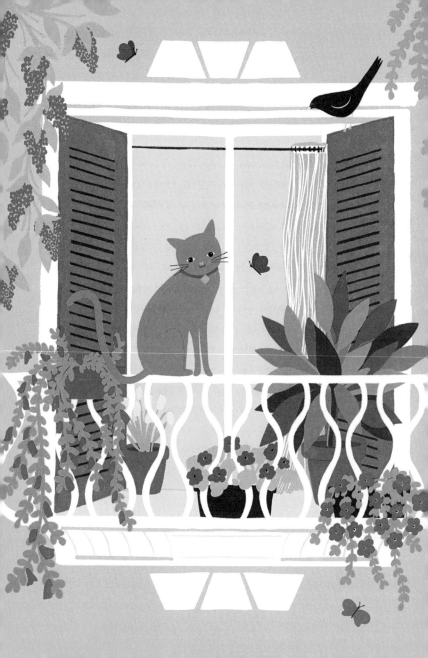

PART ONE
UNDERSTANDING YOUR CAT

Just as it does in humans, the chakra system holds the key to so many imbalances in our feline companions, whether they are of a physical, emotional or spiritual nature. By unlocking these imbalances, we not only enable our cats to live in greater comfort and joy, but we can unravel their untold stories – sometimes even more effectively than through animal communication. By taking a deeper dive into energy fields and discovering the positive effects of chakra balancing, we can learn so much more about ourselves and our feline companions.

An additional benefit of chakra balancing in animals is that the healing journey is often mutual – so we can heal ourselves as we heal them. Thus, we work together towards knowledge, healing and growth while deepening our bonds with one another.

THE PSYCHIC CONNECTION

You are psychic – and you have a psychic connection with your cat! Did you know that? Perhaps without even thinking about it, you somehow know how your cat feels, what she wants or needs and possibly even her innermost thoughts. This goes beyond simply reading the normal body language of your feline friend or her subtle nuances to the deep connection the two of you share. You may not be fully conscious of it, but on some level, you just know; your spiritual lives are intertwined.

If some or all of this doesn't resonate with you just yet, don't let it concern you. It's something that will develop naturally and by osmosis – and with a little intention, focus and what you're about to learn from this book thrown in. I would bet that even if you are not aware of it, you've already begun to connect with your feline companion. Conversely, your cat also knows the true inner you: your deepest thoughts, feelings, needs and desires. And this goes beyond the invisible stuff like feelings and emotions, carrying through to the material plane and anything that is going on within your physical body. So how is that possible and how does this work?

Each of us (both us and our feline friends) has an aura – a field of energy surrounding our physical bodies (which you'll learn about later). When we spend time with one another, our energy fields naturally intermingle and share space. It's in this place and time that we become familiar with and absorb energies from each other. This is the entry point into the way we "read" one another and our ailments as well as sharing information and even types of communication. Our cats love to share space and energy with us, and if you happen to be a healer or are training to be one, you will surely know how drawn your furry feline is to any form of healing, energy or spiritual work.

If you don't yet have experience with healing, not to worry. Anyone can learn to heal cats, and likewise, your cat can heal you too. This place of mutual healing begins with the basics of connecting and communicating with your feline companion. That shared space of your energy fields and the connection you already have with your furry friend is a great place to start – and the psychic link can open up a deeper level of communication that further strengthens your bond.

Tuning in to your cat on a deeper level will allow you to learn anything your cat might want you to know – they can be small things, or bigger, more important things. It will give you a greater insight into your cat's overall wellbeing, including information related to the physical, emotional, mental and even spiritual aspects. Yes, your cat is a spiritual being!

There are a few methods by which we learn more about our cats on a deeper level, and the more we practise, the easier it will become. Sometimes we may sense what our cat is experiencing; other times we may learn by seeing, feeling, hearing or simply knowing. At other times, we may need to tune in deliberately and actively in order to determine our cat's wellbeing and current state, or anything else our cats want to communicate to us.

Communication through Imaging

If you try communicating with your feline friend and don't feel as if it is working right away, don't give up. This skill can take time to develop, and it can depend on your openness, past training and current level of experience. However, one of the most important things you can do for success in connection and healing is to quieten your mind, especially any negative inner voices that may rear their ugly heads. Disruptive thoughts or distractions can muddy the psychic link and may prevent you from receiving communication clearly. Since our connections with our feline friends can often manifest in the form of images, if you feel stumped about what your cat is trying to tell you, it can help to imagine what that might be. Then go with whatever pops into your head first, as imagination is simply "imaging". This helps to prime the pump for a greater connection and further opening in communication.

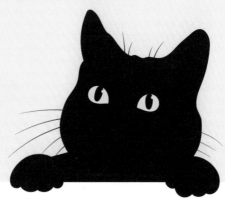

Connecting Energy Fields

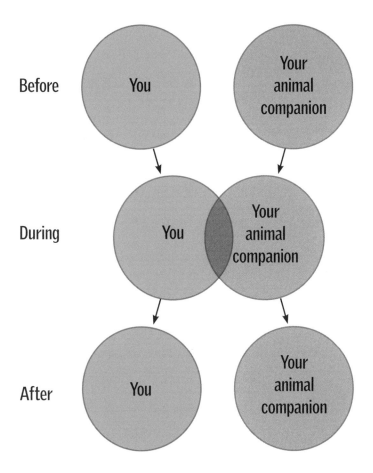

Before · During · After

Connecting Energies

 Create a space as free from noise and distraction as possible where you can relax, undisturbed, and refer to the diagram on page 13.

 To begin with, uncross your arms and legs, straighten your back, and bring yourself into a relaxed and comfortable position – either sitting or lying down.

 Close your eyes if you are in a position to do so. Take a couple of deep breaths, inhaling through the nose and exhaling through the mouth. As you breathe in, visualize breathing in universal white light healing energy and exhaling any worries, fears or doubts you may have.

 Now, visualize your energy field or aura as an orb around you that encompasses your physical body plus an extra 3–6 ft (1–2 m) around you.

 Next, I'd like you to visualize your cat and visualize their energy field or aura as an orb around them. This orb encompasses their physical body plus an extra 1–2 ft (30–60 cm), depending on their size.

Now, in your mind's eye, visualize two energy fields (yours and theirs) as similar-sized circles in front of you (see page 13).

 Have them move together until a portion of each is overlapping. This portion will make up roughly one-third of each energy field; this is the place where your energy fields come together, and you connect.

 Notice how you feel when connected to your furry friend.

 See if you receive any impressions – thoughts, feelings, colours, images or messages – and make a note of them.

 When you are ready, visualize or think of the two energy fields moving apart from one another so there is no longer an overlap, and each field is left separate and whole. Disconnecting is good energy hygiene, so neither is left energetically burdened by the other.

 Open your eyes and return to the present, knowing that you have made an important step in linking up with your cat.

Be receptive to anything your cat might send your way and take notice of everything you pick up. Even if it feels unconventional, uncomfortable or unexpected – or if you think it may have come from you – don't discount it. Sometimes the most subtle of communications can seem like our own thoughts, but it's important to pay attention to everything you receive, even if it doesn't make sense straight away. You might even receive short "lightning" bursts of information, feelings, sensations or energy; these are especially important to take note of. Picture your mind as an empty canvas or a blank book, ready to receive, and then allow the page to fill with your cat's message. The more open you are to the connection, the more you will receive, and the more receptive you will be to assessing and healing your feline companion.

The gift of connecting psychically with our cats is an innate one, and acknowledging the psychic link and trusting your own intuition are vital in the connection process. Your instinct is there for a reason, and it can help guide you through connecting and communicating with your cat. This often requires some level of letting go, especially of doubts, expectations and control. Attempts at connection may not go the way you might expect; allow the process to flow naturally. This will create and strengthen a psychic link that is clean and pure, providing a foundation for clearer, stronger connection and bonding. Trust your cat and your connection, and follow it wherever it leads.

If you feel like anything is blocking your connection, take some time to visualize letting go of that blockage and shift your focus to the energy field connection you share with your cat.

Clearing a Blockage

To clear a blockage in your connection to your cat, try the following exercise.

 Visualize a physical representation of the blockage, then watch it turn to dust, fall to the ground and be swept away.

 Next, picture the connection between your heart and brow chakras to the heart chakra of your cat, and allow your energy fields to mingle (see page 19).

 You can even visualize your energy fields coming together and overlapping, and then stay receptive to see what you sense or feel.

(We will cover energy fields more in depth in the next section, so don't worry if you feel like you need more information.)

As humans, it can take some time to get used to opening the psychic link with our feline companions. Have patience with yourself and keep practising. Your cat is already open and is sharing with you and her feline friends naturally; it's second nature to her. But it's us who have to take the leap and often stretch ourselves outside of our comfort zones to awaken these innate gifts and abilities that allow us to receive the information. Once you establish the psychic connection with your cat from your perspective, it will always be there for you, and you will find it becomes easier to reconnect from there on out.

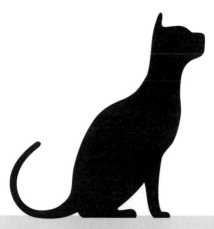

 TIP: Remember to stay calm and focused, set your intention, be open to whatever comes your way, and you'll undoubtedly feel a closer connection to your feline companion in no time.

Jiggs' Telepathic Pyramid

The image shows your connection (or psychic link) with your cat.

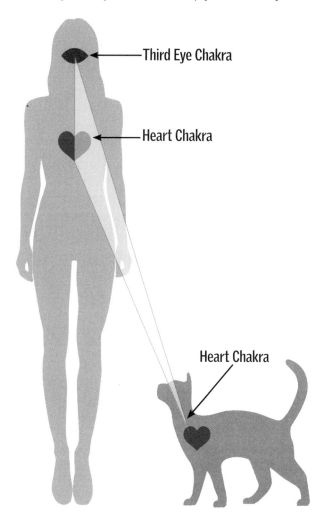

Third Eye Chakra

Heart Chakra

Heart Chakra

THE ENERGY FIELD

To learn about the chakras, first it is important to have a general understanding of the entire energy field – or energy body, as it's often called – and a knowledge of the way it works. The energy field is an invisible but vital component of any living being, and much like ours, our feline companion's energy field is comprised of three major components: the aura, the meridians and the chakras.

The Subtle Bodies or Aura

The aura is comprised of various layers of energy bodies, often called subtle bodies. Subtle bodies are layers of energy surrounding your feline companion's body, similar to a Russian doll. The physical body makes up the innermost layer, followed by the etheric double, the emotional body and the spiritual body. The image opposite shows a cat's aura and various layers of subtle bodies.

The Subtle Bodies

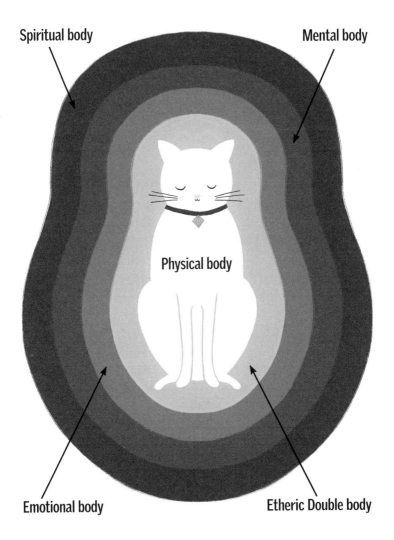

Spiritual body

Mental body

Physical body

Emotional body

Etheric Double body

Meridians

A concept in traditional Chinese medicine that has become mainstream during more recent times, meridians are pathways through which life force energy flows. In very simplistic terms, you can think of meridians as etheric veins running throughout your cat's body, through which energy is transported. Studies have been done to prove that the vital organs and bodily systems rely on this energy as they rely on food, blood and air to survive.

Chakras

Chakras are energy vortexes, or portals, located in various spots throughout the body. Spinning and emanating outwards, chakras are vehicles for the assimilation of vital life force energy. This life force energy is filtered into a cat through their chakras and then through their entire being. When there are imbalances or blockages, these can inhibit assimilation, resulting in physical, emotional or behavioural symptoms. It's important to note that chakras are like cones, originating at points on the midline of the body, like stems, and fanning outwards through each of the layers of the subtle body.

To make things simple, if this concept is new to you, you can compare the subtle body, or aura, to the physical body; the chakras to the organs; and the meridians to the veins. This is a very basic approach, but it may help beginners to remember the different parts of the energy field.

Let's delve a little deeper into chakras. The word "chakra" is a Sanskrit word meaning "wheel", and the chakras are often referred to as "wheels of light" or "wheels of life". The concept originated in India over 4,000 years ago, and chakras are commonly referred to today in yoga and healing practices.

Chakras tell a story

Chakras can be regarded as "maps of consciousness" of an individual being, as they can tell the story of what has taken place in the experience and life of a cat – from surgeries to traumas and emotional upsets. It is where our feline companions receive energetic sustenance. All vital life force energy is filtered into an animal's energetic body through these portals, the chakras, and is then funnelled via the meridians into the endocrine system (which consists of various glands). This is how it ends up impacting our feline friends on a physical level. The degree to which their chakras are healthy, balanced and whole plays a large part in the way this life force energy reaches and enriches them.

There are numerous vortexes of energy within your cat that can be called chakras. However, it is the nine major and thirteen minor chakras, which correlate with various states of health, wellbeing and consciousness, that we are going to concern ourselves with. Chakras can be seen or felt (by some) as spinning wheels of energy and resemble cones, with both a front and a back side, spinning in opposite directions. Think of the way you squeeze out a wet towel, with one hand twisting one way and the other hand twisting the other; this is similar to the way chakras flow.

The Chakra Vortex

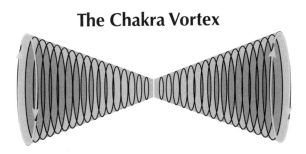

How Energy Flows to Our Felines

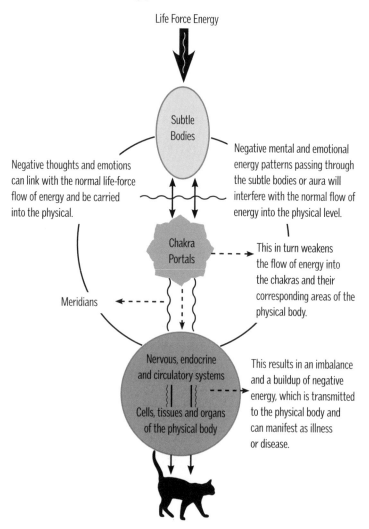

Life Force Energy

Subtle Bodies

Negative thoughts and emotions can link with the normal life-force flow of energy and be carried into the physical.

Negative mental and emotional energy patterns passing through the subtle bodies or aura will interfere with the normal flow of energy into the physical level.

Chakra Portals

This in turn weakens the flow of energy into the chakras and their corresponding areas of the physical body.

Meridians

Nervous, endocrine and circulatory systems

Cells, tissues and organs of the physical body

This results in an imbalance and a buildup of negative energy, which is transmitted to the physical body and can manifest as illness or disease.

Chakra anatomy

Chakras vary in brightness, depth and size, from strong to weak, and also in the amount of energy, depending upon the health and vitality of your feline friend. Each chakra governs different glands and organs in the physical body, and each also relates to specific emotional, mental and spiritual aspects of consciousness. An animal's thoughts and feelings also filter through the chakras, eventually resulting in manifestations that show up in the physical body.

When energy does not flow freely in the chakras, your cat's body is not able to function properly. Stress of any kind – whether of a physical, emotional, mental or spiritual nature – can cause an imbalance in our animal companion's chakras. This imbalance can eventually lead to disease if it is not cleared and balanced.

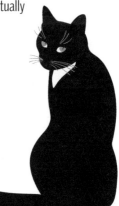

 TIP: It is important to remember that a situation or event that stresses one individual may not stress another, as some beings are much more sensitive than others.

Healing

We can alter the chakras through healing. It is also possible for other influences to alter them (in both positive and negative ways). It does not require any special talents for you to learn to heal your feline companions through their chakras – just a strong desire to do so and the intention to understand and help them. For some of you, simply using the chakra charts included in this book and placing your hands in the area of each chakra will be enough. You can also feel for the energy vortex or energy spin, and as you become accustomed to the feel of the chakras – and particularly your cat's chakras, as each is different – you may start to feel or sense whether they are balanced or not.

Locating the chakras

Please note that not all people will be able to see or feel their cat's chakras. Over time, and with practice, most of us will be able to locate them in one way or another. If you're having difficulty, don't be discouraged; just maintain your trust and focus on what you intend to do, and use the chart provided as a guide. Either way, you can still perform beneficial healing and clearing work for your cat from wherever you are currently.

Ways to Find
the Chakras

Seeing: Actually seeing energy moving
or colour present in a chakra.

🐾

Feeling: Feeling definitive movement of
energy in the area of a chakra.

🐾

Sensing: Using your inner knowing and
guidance to determine where a chakra is located.

🐾

Dowsing: Using pendulum dowsing (if you know how)
to detect where a chakra is.

🐾

Kinesiology: Using muscle testing (if you know how)
to detect the location of a chakra.

**We'll talk more about this and how to balance your cat's
chakras in Part Two.**

WORKING WITH CATS

Whether your cat is a kitten, elderly or a mature adult cat in her prime, we approach chakra (and other) healing work the same way for each individual. Unfortunately, in today's world, there are many cats who have been subject to abuse, trauma, abandonment, the rescue system and more, as well as feral cats, who have had little to no interaction with humans and who are completely undomesticated. Most of you will probably be applying the practices you learn in this book to help your own domesticated cats, but you can also take the skills you learn here and help to heal any cat, including rescued and feral cats – either those still living in the wild, those who have been taken in under a spay, neuter and release programme, or those who have been rehomed so they can live a happier and more comfortable life. Cats and kittens who have been rescued, abused, traumatized or abandoned require special concessions when it comes to healing.

Signs Your Cat Is Unwell

Always contact your veterinarian if you notice any changes in your cat, whether physical or behavioural. Watch for changes in her eating, drinking, digestion and litter box habits as well as notable mood or other normal routine changes. Issues such as excessive hunger, refusing to eat, vomiting, diarrhea, constipation, hair loss, sudden bad breath, eye or nose discharge, pupil dilation, wounds or swelling, over- or under-grooming, lethargy or hiding from you should always be considered signs of potential illness until otherwise ruled out.

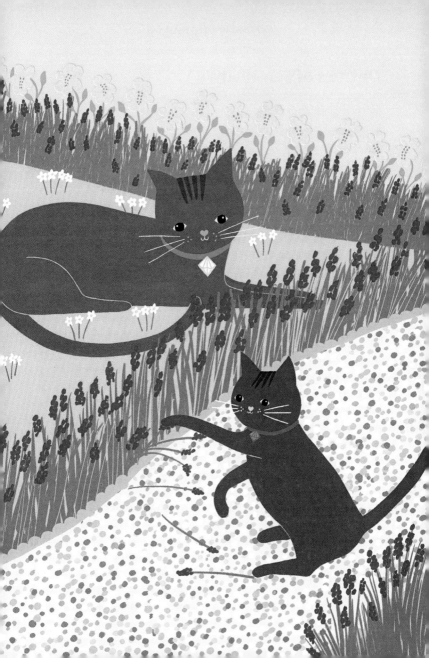

Degrees of Sensitivity

Before beginning any healing work on your cat, always take stock of how delicate an otherwise healthy cat or kitten might be – physically, emotionally and mentally – as this will vary from being to being. Think of cats as falling into categories of low, medium and high sensitivity.

Low sensitivity: A large proportion of domesticated cats fall into this category, particularly those who live with families and are used to noise and regular handling.

Medium sensitivity: I consider a kitten, elderly cat or a cat who has just had surgery to be much more delicate than average, so I'd place them in this group.

High sensitivity: I would place abused, traumatized, abandoned, rescued and feral cats in this group as they are often profoundly frightened, shocked and sometimes even terrified.

These are generalizations, of course, and as with all generalizations, there are exceptions to the rule. For the new healer, having these three categories is a good place to start, and as cats are living beings, we would rather have you err on the side of caution of a cat having more sensitivity rather than less.

The fact that cats are in general one of the most sensitive of the domesticated species, especially when it comes to energy and healing work, should always be carefully considered when working with them. One of the first rules of healing is to do no harm, and this includes never allowing your healing work to create additional stress in a cat. It is intended only to alleviate stress and tension and bring forth greater wellbeing.

Hands-on or Distance Healing

While some cats may enjoy a hands-on approach to chakra healing and balancing, many others will much prefer a hands-off method. This can be related to their specific sensitivity grouping mentioned earlier, with the more delicate ones being inclined to prefer distance work (but it's not always that way). Whether you're working hands-on or hands-off, your results should not vary. Performing hands-off or distance healing on your cat simply means conducting the healing method anywhere from a few feet to a continent away. This approach is just as effective and provides the same results you would get by working hands-on.

Preparing Your Cat for Chakra Work

Everything in this Universe is energy and our feline friends are impacted by all of it – much more than you might expect. Cats act as sponges for us, helping clear our energy, and they are also susceptible to their own imbalances. Aside from their own issues, the thoughts, feelings, mindsets and illnesses of those around them, planetary energies, injustices to their species as a whole, and even global energies like pandemics and wars impact them and can create imbalances. Because of this, healing is very beneficial for your cat, as it helps her to release all this unwanted, non-beneficial energy. The first step I recommend when preparing to work with your cat is to ground and protect her.

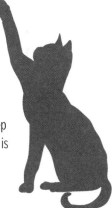

Please note, the following exercise can be done physically on the body, in the aura (about 4–6 in/10–15 cm above her body), or over distance – from across a room or even in another location. Always honour what your feline companion prefers. Sensitive animals generally prefer it to be performed off the body. If your feline friend has touchy paws, you can do the exercise hands-on, but then hold your hands above the paws when you get to that area. Our main goal is healing, so we don't want to add any extra stress.

If you are familiar with energy fields, as you're performing this exercise, visualize and set the intention that your cat's chakras, subtle bodies and meridians will come into perfect balance each time you do it.

As with ours, the energy field of animals can become imbalanced through stressors, the environment, shock, trauma and absorbing energy from others. This simple grounding exercise is designed to reconnect them with the energy of Mother Earth, which is the most natural state for any living being.

Grounding Your Cat's Energy

This exercise consists of a series of three strokes.

 To begin, bring yourself into a calm, focused state; take a few deep, cleansing breaths, releasing any stresses of the day.

 With the middle and index finger of each hand together (with the sides of each index finger touching), trace a line from the tip of your cat's nose up the middle of the face, between the eyes and ears, along the midline of the body (spine) to the shoulders, then separate your hands and bring one hand down each shoulder and leg to the top of her front paws. As you're doing this, visualize your cat's energy flowing along with it. At the paws, rest gently and visualize her energy going down through the floor and into the ground below, connecting deep with Mother Earth and releasing any non-beneficial energy. Let your cat or your intuition tell you how long to hold – generally between 30 seconds and two minutes – until you feel her energy connecting deep within the Earth.

Repeat that stroke, but this time, go all the way to her hips before separating your hands and tracing down each back leg, as you did with the front legs in the first stroke. Again, visualize your cat's energy flowing along with the stroke and her energy going into the ground below, connecting deeply with Mother Earth. Hold for a time as before.

Finally, repeat this once more, but go all the way to the tail and trace along to the tail tip (or what would have been the tail tip in an animal with a docked tail) and cup your hands there and hold, allowing for her energy to go down into the ground and connect her deeply with Mother Earth.

When you have finished, visualize your cat's aura in a protective bubble of pink light (pink is for healing). The bubble should be permeable to loving energies and repel non-beneficial energies. To help this transpire, visualize hearts (as loving energies) coming towards the protective bubble of pink light surrounding your cat and permeating the bubble. Then visualize arrows (as non-beneficial energies) coming towards the protective bubble of pink light surrounding your cat and being repelled by the bubble.

HEALING PRINCIPLES

The principles of healing are underpinned by beliefs, intentions and wishes – our own and those of our companions – and our commitment to our work.

Our Beliefs

We believe that felines are sacred beings, just like all other beings, and that they have divine wisdom to share with us. We feel that they are in our lives for connection and healing as well as teaching and guidance.

We understand that through connection and communication, our cats can help heal us and we can heal them. By building strong relationships with our cats that transcend the physical plane, we are awakened to the deep connection we share. We recognize that felines help us navigate the circle of life and guide us throughout our existence in many ways.

Our cats possess multiple levels of consciousness – physical, emotional, mental and spiritual – that allow us access for connection, communication and healing. We respect the sacredness of each of our cats and listen intuitively to their responses, proceeding with the utmost care and respect.

We also respect our cat's wishes for healing and honour her preference for hands-on or distance techniques as desired. We release any judgements about the connection, communication, and healing of our feline friend and trust that her higher self, and our open heart, will lead us to a place of true healing for both of us.

Our Commitment

We commit to partnering with our feline friends and asking permission before beginning any connection or healing work. We draw upon our connection with our cat and work towards healing with an open mind, allowing her to guide her own journey for the highest good of all involved. We also commit to deferring to the expertise of a veterinary professional when necessary to diagnose any condition or ailment.

We commit to practising and fostering our own spiritual growth and self-healing in order to be a clear and strong channel for harmonious connection and restorative energy healing with our cats. We trust our own hearts and wisdom and try our best to avoid allowing emotions to cloud our judgements or diminish our connection.

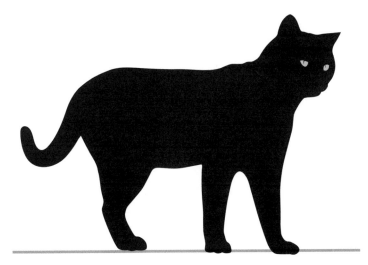

HEALING MODALITIES

The way we prepare ourselves to perform our healing work is just as important as the healing techniques themselves.

Ourselves as Conduits

When it comes to healing, it is important to recognize we are simply the conduits for the healing to take place; we are not the ones causing it. It is God, the Universe, or whatever higher power you subscribe to that creates and determines the final healing result. We always do our very best with the highest intention to help any living being, but if a being doesn't heal the way we envisioned, it's beyond our control and not our fault. I always ask that the healing be in accordance with divine order and for the "highest and best good" of the cat and all concerned, as there may be prior spiritual agreements or contracts at play. This never stops us from trying, though, as even in the death and dying process, healing work can be beneficial to your cat and healing can be received.

Preparing Ourselves for Chakra Work

When performing healing work, it's important to place ourselves into what is known as a "healing state". It's a peaceful state, similar to a meditative state, but where we're a little more alert and aware. Being in this state is as important (or even more so) than the accuracy of the healing techniques we perform.

Preparing for Healing Work

For best results:

Relax

❖

Intensify your focus

❖

Quiet any distracting mind chatter

❖

Enter a peaceful, grounded and centred state

❖

Adopt an unobtrusive energy resonance that creates an opening and space
for the cat to come to you (physically or energetically)

❖

Set aside your ego mind

❖

Move into your heart centre

❖

Be highly respectful and non-judgemental

❖

Ask the permission of the cat being you are about to work with

Setting Your Intention

Another important component is your intention; it's as important as the technique you employ when it comes to healing your fur friend. When you work on your cat's chakras, I recommend creating an intention for the end result of the healing work you do. Here are a couple of examples of what I mean:

"I intend that Pixie Rose's inflammation and pain be eliminated."

"I intend to help Phoebe adapt to the houseguests we'll be having next week."

"I intend that Tulip's spay surgery takes place smoothly and without incident."

"I intend that Sheba's transition to the spirit realm happens smoothly and peacefully."

You can ask for anything when it comes to healing, whether it's a physical, emotional, mental or spiritual result; no goal or dream is too big. Even if your cat has an incurable or life-threatening disease, it doesn't hurt to ask for healing, as I've seen many miracles in my 30-plus years of doing this work. At the end of my intention, I always like to say, "I ask for this or something better, so be it."

Visualization

Visualization is another powerful healing tool. You can visualize the chakras, visualize which ones require balancing and visualize them coming into perfect balance. You will also use visualization in some of the other balancing tools.

Your Healing Team

Each of us has a team of benevolent beings that are willing and want to help us in our healing work. Mostly, they are beings who have already crossed over: ancestors, elders, loved ones – both human and animal – and even well-known beings like the patron saint of animals, St Francis of Assisi, or the clairvoyant Edgar Cayce. You don't have to know your healing team intimately, but I urge you to call them in to be with you when working on your cat.

Hands-on Healing

As the name implies, hands-on healing is done by placing your hands on or immediately above the body, in this case the chakra, and intending that universal healing energy flows to the animal and corrects any imbalance.

Distance Healing

Distance healing can be done anywhere, from a few feet to a continent away from the animal, while intending that universal healing energy flows to the animal and corrects any imbalance.

If you currently share your life with a feline friend, the chances are that you know her well enough to know whether she would prefer a hands-on or hands-off approach – but if not, just try each method and let her enthusiasm for and reaction to each tell you which one she prefers. A hands-off approach is preferred by many felines.

Sensing Your Cat's Chakras

 Once you're in a healing state, use the diagram on pages 52–3 to locate each of the chakras on your cat's body.

 Then, using your fingertips, start about 4–6 in (10–15 cm) above the body in the general area of each chakra, and slowly lower your finger towards your cat's body at the chakra point. You can work in their energy field or directly on the body (more on this below). Determine, one by one, if you see (with your physical eyes or in your mind's eye), hear, feel or sense anything; some of you will and some of you won't, and all are equally fine.

 If working hands-on, it's okay to hold your hand directly on your cat's body and continue feeling and sensing, as long as she is not in any way irritated or agitated by it. Some highly sensitive cats will find this to be too much pressure, energetically speaking, even if you're barely touching her – so be sure to honour this. Some people will feel the chakra energy as a buzzing or tingling, as heat or cold or another sensation, even if it's very subtle – while others may have to work at it and practise over time to sensitize themselves to this subtle energy.

Determining Which of Your Cat's Chakras Is Out of Balance

Using the exercise opposite, you may be able to feel a subtle difference in your cat's chakras. Some chakras will feel like they are in perfect balance, while others may feel out of balance. Again, this may take some time and practise to determine. If you happen to know how to do muscle testing or dowsing, you can use either of these methods to determine or confirm which of your cat's chakras need balancing. You can also simply ask to be shown or told which chakras most need healing. The latter requires trust in your psychic/intuitive abilities.

If none of these options seems feasible to you, you can simply use the information provided in Part Two of this book to work on the chakra most relevant to your cat's symptoms, behaviours or conditions, or you can work on each of them in turn.

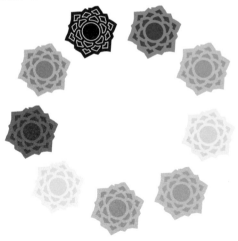

Balancing the Chakras

You can bring your cat's chakras into balance, one by one, by simply using a strong intention to do so while holding your hand over each chakra you are intending to balance. Then wait until it happens and until you feel it is complete. Becoming proficient at this requires lots of trust and a big leap of faith.

Another way to do this, and the one I use most frequently, is simply by using the healing statement I've included for each chakra. Here's an example:

> **"I send red light to [cat's name]'s root chakra and ask that it come into perfect balance, spinning in an appropriate fashion, with any imbalances, blockages or non-beneficial energies being released to the spiritual. And so it is."**

In this example, I used the colour (red) that is associated with the particular chakra I was balancing (the root chakra). To use this process for the chakras you intend to balance for your cat, see the information listed for each chakra in Part Two of this book.

You can also work with your cat's chakras using a variety of other methods, including:

Spirit animals

This is a more shamanic approach; each chakra has a related spirit animal. You can call in the spirit of the corresponding animal to come to your feline friend to heal, balance and clear her chakras and any and all related conditions.

Physical stimulation

Weak chakras can be stimulated physically with various activities such as exercise, bathing or massage, depending on the particular chakra you are working on. Obviously, most cats strongly dislike baths so bathing is not generally an option.

Archangels

Call in the archangel related to each chakra to come to your cat and assist with balance and clearing her chakras and any and all related conditions.

Affirmations

Use the affirmations provided for each chakra as they apply to your cat (be sure to customize them).

Visualization

Visualize the chakra in its current state, and then the way you'd like it to be. Then, on the count of three, visualize it coming into perfect balance. Then set the intention that it will "lock in" to this balanced fashion and remain balanced.

Sending frequencies

Radionics, as it is known, is a technique that is conducted to send particularly restorative energetic frequencies to your cat for the purposes of promoting healing, and in this case, healing of a specific chakra. This can be done with a radionics machine or through your own intention and energy. If this topic interests you, I suggest further study. But for the sake of simplicity here, use the Sending Frequencies exercise on the next page.

Sending Frequencies

 Once you are in your healing state, you can send frequencies to your cat using the following statement along with a strong intention:

> "I send [substance] to [cat's name] and ask that she receive it perfectly now, on all levels, all dimensions, all aspects, known and unknown, now and for all time."

 Then visualize and intend that it is being received by your cat for as long as it is in her highest and best good. You can use this method to send crystals, colours or flower essences/gem elixirs, etc. to your cat.

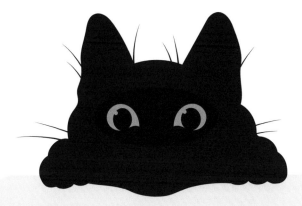

Examples of Sending Frequencies

"I send smoky quartz to Bella and ask that she receive it perfectly now, on all levels, all dimensions, as aspects, known and unknown, now and for all time."

"I send the colour turquoise to Willow and ask that she receive it perfectly now, on all levels, all dimensions, as aspects, known and unknown, now and for all time."

"I send Bach Rescue Remedy to Petunia and ask that she receive it perfectly now, on all levels, all dimensions, as aspects, known and unknown, now and for all time."

Pendulum Dowsing or Muscle Testing

If you know how to pendulum dowse or muscle test to determine which chakras most need balancing, you can employ these methods in your chakra work. If you are not well-versed in dowsing, we will cover it in more depth in Part Three, so I recommend you wait until then to work with chakras in this way. If you are familiar with muscle testing, feel free to apply it using whatever method you choose. See the exercise opposite.

Alternatively, you could dowse or muscle test the percentage (the score out of 100) for each of your cat's chakras, and when you're done, you can work on your cat's three lowest values. If you have a tie for your cat's third lowest-scoring chakra, then simply work with her four lowest-scoring chakras.

Brain Integration

Brain integration balances the right and left hemispheres of the brain. Trace a figure eight over the area of the chakra you want to balance for your cat, in her aura, with the intention of harmonizing the energy and bringing it into perfect balance. Visualize a number "8" on its side, like an infinity symbol but with more rounded loops; then, with the palm of your hand, trace the sideways eight beginning in the centre, at the "X" (or where it crosses over). From the centre, come down to the left and up and around and cross the middle, then down to the right and up and around and cross the middle. Trace this pattern three to five times, first in the direction of the chakra you wish to balance, and then in the direction of the entire energy field.

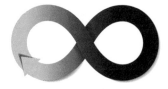

Determining Priority Chakras

You can use a pendulum to determine which chakra most needs balancing (the priority chakra, as I call it), and to help you do the actual balancing.

 Use "yes" or "no" questions and follow a line of questioning like this for the major chakras:

"Is [cat's name]'s lowest-scoring chakra the root chakra?"
If no, your next question would be:

"Is [cat's name]'s lowest-scoring chakra the sexual progression chakra?" If no, your next question would be:

"Is [cat's name]'s lowest-scoring chakra the solar plexus chakra?", and continue these questions for each of the nine major chakras (see pages 52–3).

 Next, you would do the same to find your cat's second and third lowest-scoring chakras until you have all three.

 Once you have determined your cat's lowest-scoring chakra (let's say it's the sensing chakra), take a pendulum, hold it over her sensing chakra and spin it to the right, while at the same time asking that her sensing chakra come into perfect balance "with any imbalances, blockages or non-beneficial energies to be released to the spiritual".

 Give the chakra some time to begin to resonate with the swing of the pendulum. Then, after 30–90 seconds, you can again use your pendulum or muscle testing technique to recheck the chakra. This time, it should be in perfect balance.

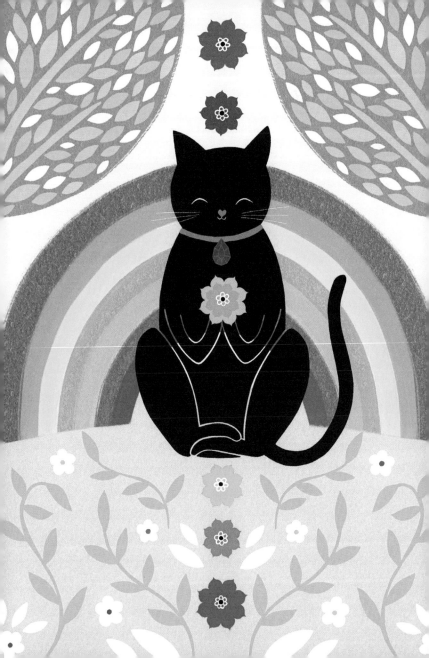

PART TWO
THE CHAKRAS

Each of your cat's chakras governs and relates to key qualities, areas, matters, issues, bodily systems, organs and emotions. Cats have both major and minor chakras, with some of the major chakras being stand-alone chakras and others having associated minor chakras. For example, in the case of one of the major chakras, the sensing chakra, there are a number of related minor or sub-chakras that are associated with it and which relate specifically to certain detailed components of it. The minor chakras associated with the sensing chakra are the following: the paw pads, the whiskers, the eyes, the ears, the nose and the tip of the tail. We will explore the major chakras first and then delve into the minor chakras.

THE MAJOR CHAKRAS

The health, wellbeing and balance of any chakra is impacted by life experiences. This can include anything and everything that occurs from the time of conception and birth right through to the present moment in the lives of each cat, and it can also include past life issues. Because of this, kittens and cats who have been through accidents, traumas, illnesses, surgeries, abuse, homelessness, kitten farms, etc., will almost always require more chakra clearing.

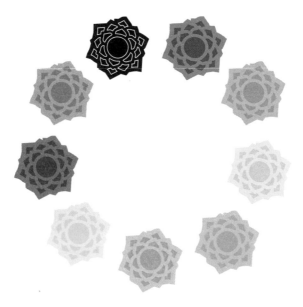

A cat can have a chakra that is out of balance with only one of the associated traits listed in the sections that follow being obvious to you, and sometimes even without any of the associated traits apparently present. Remember, matters of a physical, emotional, mental or spiritual nature can all impact a chakra – but not all are required for an imbalance to be present. Energy is a complex and vast topic, and the way it works and impacts our feline companions is not always linear. Be sure to trust your findings and balance her chakras whether you understand why they are out of balance or not.

Issues in our felines can impact more than one chakra, and healing them often crosses over to a number of chakras. Thus, don't be surprised if more than one is out of balance for your cat as a result of one issue or area of concern.

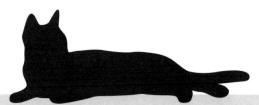

 Chakra healing is a wonderful complementary treatment but never delay veterinary care or try to heal medical conditions solely on your own.

The Nine Major Chakra Points

Like us, your cat's body is not just physical; it's made up of energy and the chakras are the major energy centres, or vortexes, that aid in the absorption and distribution of that energy.

Working with your cat's chakras to get them balanced, flowing and in harmony can keep her at peak health and wellness and allow her to recover from any physical or emotional trauma. Unlike us, cats have an extra major chakra, the brachial (see pages 86–9).

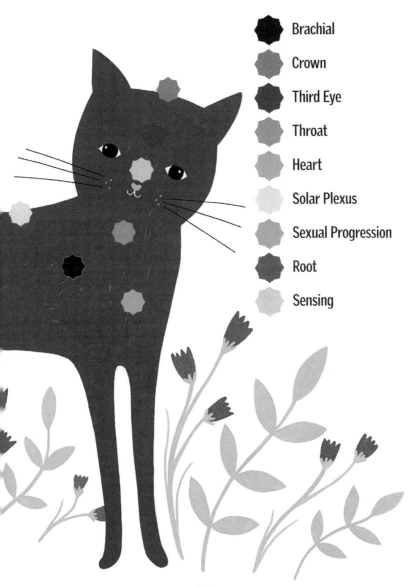

- Brachial
- Crown
- Third Eye
- Throat
- Heart
- Solar Plexus
- Sexual Progression
- Root
- Sensing

53

Root Chakra
(Base Chakra)

The root chakra is related to issues of the physical world, health, strength, stability, nourishment, boundaries, self-preservation, survival instinct, feeling comfortable in their skin, feeling grounded and status in a family or clan (this includes the human and animal family – of both cats and other species). Generational and early life wounds are found in this chakra, as well as energies related to the species as a whole. Connected to matters of safety, courage individuality, security, patience and instincts such as the fight-or-flight response.

Location: The root chakra is located at the coccyx, or base of the tail.

Associated colours: Red, coral red or sometimes black.

Associated glands/organs: Adrenals, kidneys, spine, colon, anus, hips, legs and paws, bones, blood.

Possible imbalance: Insecurity, fear, lack of trust, anxiety, arthritis, incontinence, territorial aggression, inappropriate scratching, blood issues, orthopaedic issues, kidney (renal) disease, hip dysplasia, constipation, diarrhoea, anal gland issues, IBS or IBD, feline immunodeficiency virus (FIV), feline leukaemia virus (FeLV).

🐾 A balanced root chakra can result in a cat who is in good health, vital, comfortable in her body, has a sense of trust in her world, feels safe and secure, has the ability to relax and be still, is stable, flourishing, generous and enjoys her role.

🐾 An imbalanced root chakra can result in a cat who is fearful, distrusting, aggressive, fails to thrive, is timid, hyperactive, stingy, jealous and is fearful of missing out, wanting more.

Spirit animal: The spirit or totem animal associated with the root chakra is the horse. The horse relates to courage, strength and stability. Call in or ask horse energy to come forth to your feline companion to be with her for the purpose of healing her root chakra.

Ways to stimulate the root chakra: Conduct a grounding exercise for your cat (see pages 32–3), give your cat a full-body massage or touch her gently all over to help her to connect better with her various body parts. Encourage exercise, stretching and scratching (a post).

Archangel: Uriel is the archangel associated with the root chakra. You can call upon Archangel Uriel to ground your cat's energy through the root chakra and at the same time to release any and all non-beneficial energies to be transmuted by the spiritual realm.

Affirmations: You can create your own affirmation to suit your cat's particular situation or use one of the following:
"[Cat's name] is happy, healthy and whole."
"[Cat's name] feels fully supported and loved."
"[Cat's name] trusts herself and her surroundings."

Visualization: If you've determined that the root chakra is imbalanced, first visualize it as it currently is, and then, on the count of three, visualize it coming into perfect balance. Then visualize "locking it in" to this balanced fashion so that it will stay balanced.

Colour therapy: Physically apply the colour red to the root chakra as well as to the rest of the body. This can be done by laying red fabric on the body, a piece of red fabric over your cat's bed, bathing your cat in red light from a light bulb covered in a red theatrical colour gel (do not shine this directly in your cat's eyes, though, as this may counteract the healing process in some sensitive beings). You can also provide red-coloured toys as well as red food and water bowls.

Crystal healing: There are a number of ways to work with crystals to help balance your cat's chakras. You can send the energetic frequency of a crystal to your cat; use a crystal physically on the body via a crystal massage, aura massage or simple touch; or place the crystal in an area your cat spends a lot of time, like under a cat bed or a chair cushion.

Pendulum dowsing: If you have already determined that your cat's root chakra is imbalanced, you can take a pendulum, and while holding it over the root chakra, physically spin it to the right while at the same time asking that her chakra come into perfect balance "with any imbalances, blockages or non-beneficial energies to be released to the spiritual", as you say in the healing statement. Give it some time to begin to resonate with the swing of the pendulum. Then after a minute or two, stop and recheck the root chakra.

Brain integration: Brain integration balances the right and left hemispheres of the brain. Trace figures of eight over the area of the root chakra, in the aura of your cat with the intention of harmonizing the energy and bringing it into perfect balance. Visualize a number "8" on its side, and then with the palm of your hand, trace the sideways "8", beginning in the centre, at the "X" (or where it crosses over). From the centre, come down to the left and up and around and cross the middle, then down to the right and up and around and cross the middle. Trace this pattern three to five times, first in the direction of the root chakra and then in the direction of the entire energy field.

CRYSTALS THAT AID IN HEALING THE ROOT CHAKRA

Black tourmaline

Boji stone

Garnet

Hematite

Jet

Red jasper

Ruby

Smoky quartz

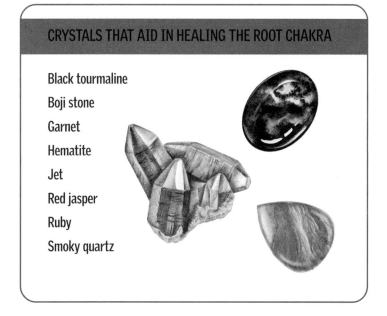

Sexual Progression Chakra
(Sacral Chakra)

Related to all aspects of procreation and sexuality, including irregular heat cycles, natural mating instinct, drive to propagate the species, spraying to mark territory, hormone imbalances, false pregnancies, mammary gland issues, inbreeding deficiencies, inherited disorders, spay and neuter issues and time spent in kitten farms. Also affects the sense of purpose, empowerment, mood, nurturing, assimilation of food, imbalanced emotions, lack of confidence, low energy, vitality and creativity.

Location: Lower abdomen to navel area.

Associated colour: Orange.

Associated glands/organs: Spleen, intestines, bladder, the internal and external male and female reproductive organs including ovaries, testicles, prostate and uterus.

Possible imbalance: Any breeding issues including infertility, spay and neuter issues and hormone imbalances (irregular heat cycles). Lack of confidence, skittishness, easily startled, hyperactive, weakness, high stress or aggression regarding cat carrier and/or car rides, cystitis, urinary tract issues, crystals, stones and blockages, low energy, lower back pain, asthma, allergies and coughs.

👣 A balanced sexual progression chakra can result in a cat who is happy, joyful, confident, empowered, relaxed, well-nourished, energized, has no issues related to the reproductive organs including spay or neuter surgeries, heat cycles or planned ethical breeding practices.

👣 An imbalanced sexual progression chakra can result in a cat who has digestive issues, is malnourished, has difficulty conceiving, experiences deficiencies from inbreeding, sprays to mark territory, is highly emotional and moody, feels unsettled at home or was abused from time spent in a kitten farm.

Spirit animal: The spirit or totem animal associated with the sexual progression chakra is the spider. The spider relates to creativity, intuition, feminine energy and the weaving of fate. Call in or ask spider energy to come forth to your feline companion to be with her for the purpose of healing her sexual progression chakra.

Ways to stimulate the sexual progression chakra: Massage (hands on the body or massage the energy field in the aura); provide your cat with a drinking fountain or trickling tap. Bathing and swimming are also options, but these are not favoured by many cats.

Archangel: Chamuel is the archangel associated with the sexual progression chakra. You can call upon Archangel Chamuel to balance your cat's energy related to the sexual progression chakra, and at the same time to release any and all non-beneficial energies to be transmuted by the spiritual realm. Feel free to list any specifics you are aware of as you ask for assistance from the archangels.

Affirmations: You can create your own affirmation to suit your cat's particular situation or use one of the following:
"[Cat's name] is at one with spay/neuter policies."
"[Cat's name] is in touch with and processes her feelings."
"[Cat's name] is well-nourished."

Visualization: If you've determined that the sexual progression chakra is imbalanced, first visualize it as it currently is, and then, on the count of three, visualize it coming into perfect balance. Then visualize "locking it in" to this balanced fashion so that it will stay balanced.

Colour therapy: Physically apply the colour orange to the sexual progression chakra as well as the rest of the body, as for the root chakra (see pages 56–7).

For crystal healing, pendulum dowsing and brain integration: Refer to these sections under the root chakra section (see pages 56–7).

CRYSTALS THAT AID IN HEALING THE SEXUAL PROGRESSION CHAKRA

Brown jasper

Carnelian

Copper citrine

Fire agate

Moonstone

Orange calcite

Orange jade

Red coral

Red quartz

Salmon

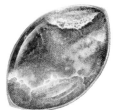

Solar Plexus Chakra

Related to issues of self-confidence, personal power and will. It affects the energetic centre of identity and personality of the cat and is considered to be one of the key centres for animals and humans to communicate physically, so it is therefore associated with how connected or disconnected a feline is to humans as well as other felines. It is also connected to predator/prey issues in cats; it takes a confident feline to hunt their prey successfully, whereas a timid one may more easily become prey for another predator. This chakra governs the sympathetic nervous system, digestive system, metabolism and emotions.

Location: Back mid-spine.

Associated colours: Yellow or gold.

Associated glands/organs: Stomach, gallbladder, pancreas, spleen, adrenals, liver, diaphragm, kidneys, nervous system, muscles.

Possible imbalance: Diabetes, digestive issues, pancreatic issues, eating issues, overweight, underweight, weight loss, excessive hunger, picky eater, food sensitivities, depression, epilepsy, hairballs, fading newborn syndrome, fears, lack of confidence, immune system issues, obsessive behaviour, training issues, nervousness, hiding, shyness, attention seeking and destructive behaviours, over-vocalization, retaliation and scratching, feline infectious peritonitis (FIP).

🐾 A balanced solar plexus chakra can result in a cat who is confident, comfortable, personable, cheerful, connected and engaged with others, experiences a well-functioning digestive system from start to finish, is calm and laid-back.

🐾 An imbalanced solar plexus chakra can result in a cat who is a picky eater; experiences vomiting, diarrhoea or constipation; lacks confidence and (sometimes) even the strength or will to live; has a weak immune system, diabetes or other metabolic issues.

Spirit animal: The spirit or totem animal associated with the solar plexus chakra is the lion. The lion relates to strength, patience, cooperation and gentleness. Call in or ask lion energy to come forth to your feline companion to be with her for the purpose of healing her solar plexus chakra.

Ways to stimulate the solar plexus chakra: Spend time with your cat in the sun or provide her with a good sunny spot; encourage her to run; while playing or offering treats, communicate with her; teach her new things.

Archangel: Jophiel is the archangel associated with the solar plexus chakra. You can call upon Archangel Jophiel to balance your cat's energy related to the solar plexus chakra, and at the same time to release any and all non-beneficial energies to be transmuted by the spiritual realm. Feel free to list any specifics you are aware of as you ask for assistance from the archangels.

Affirmations: You can create your own affirmation to suit your cat's particular situation or use one of the following:
"[Cat's name] is confident in all situations."
"[Cat's name]'s digestive system functions perfectly."
"[Cat's name] is emotionally engaged with her human and animal friends."

Visualization: If you've determined that the solar plexus chakra is imbalanced, first visualize it as it currently is, and then, on the count of three, visualize it coming into perfect balance. Then visualize "locking it in" to this balanced fashion so that it will stay balanced.

Colour therapy: Physically apply the colour yellow to the solar plexus chakra as well as the rest of the body, as for the root chakra (see pages 56–7).

For crystal healing, pendulum dowsing and brain integration: Refer to these sections under the root chakra section (see pages 56–7).

CRYSTALS THAT AID IN HEALING THE SOLAR PLEXUS CHAKRA

Amber
Citrine
Moldavite
Sunstone
Tiger Eye
Topaz
Yellow calcite
Yellow fluorite

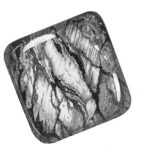

Heart Chakra

Related to both divine and unconditional love, especially the love shared between cats and their humans, but also the love shared with their animal friends as well. It is one of the places that connects cats to their higher power or source energy. A broken heart creates imbalance in this chakra, so it is a chakra that almost always needs balancing in abandoned, feral and rescue cats. It is the key area for interspecies telepathic communication (also known as animal communication) with humans, as well as communication with others – of their species and others in their household or clan. This chakra energizes the blood and physical body with life force energy.

Location: Centre of the chest, at the heart.

Associated colours: Green or pink.

Associated glands/organs: Heart, thymus, lungs, respiratory system, circulatory system, chest, immune system, front legs and paws.

Possible imbalance: Anger, aggression, broken-hearted, arthritis, anxiety, loneliness for humans or animals, heart disease, lung disease, blood disorders, emotional issues, inability to bond, respiratory infection, coughing, stress-related asthma, feline immunodeficiency virus (FIV), feline leukaemia virus (FeLV), absorbing energies, emotions, illnesses and non-beneficial energies from humans (or other animals).

🐾 A balanced heart chakra can result in a cat who has a good life, feels loved and offers love freely to both humans and other animal friends, feels energized, enjoys interspecies telepathic communication (animal communication) with her humans.

🐾 An imbalanced heart chakra can result in a cat who has a broken heart from being abandoned, feral or a part of the rescue system; has heart, respiratory or circulatory issues; is anxious, unwilling, displays anger and aggression.

Spirit animal: The spirit or totem animal associated with the heart chakra is the dolphin. The dolphin relates to love, joy, passion and fertility. Call in or ask dolphin energy to come forth to your feline companion to be with her for the purpose of healing her heart chakra.

Ways to stimulate the heart chakra: Spend time in nature; spend time watching birds, clouds or butterflies; open the windows to let the fresh air in; encourage her onto a high perch; have her spend time with loved ones.

Archangel: Raphael is the archangel associated with the heart chakra. You can call upon Archangel Raphael to balance your cat's energy related to the heart chakra, and at the same time to release any and all non-beneficial energies to be transmuted by the spiritual realm. Feel free to list any specifics you are aware of as you ask for assistance from the archangels.

Affirmations: You can create your own affirmation to suit your cat's particular situation or use one of the following:
"[Cat's name] feels all of the love sent her way."
"[Cat's name]'s negative past is released with grace and replaced with joy."
"[Cat's name]'s life force and vitality are increasing daily."

Visualization: If you've determined that the heart chakra is imbalanced, first visualize it as it currently is, and then, on the count of three, visualize it coming into perfect balance. Then visualize "locking it in" to this balanced fashion so that it will stay balanced.

Colour therapy: Physically apply the colour green or pink to the heart chakra and rest of the body, as for the root chakra (see pages 56–7).

For crystal healing, pendulum dowsing and brain integration: Refer to these sections under the root chakra section (see pages 56–7).

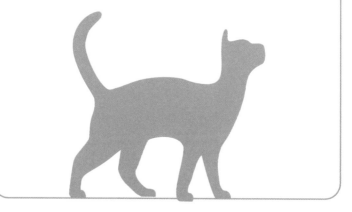

CRYSTALS THAT AID IN HEALING THE HEART CHAKRA

Aventurine

Emerald

Green quartz

Green tourmaline

Kunzite

Pink or green jade

Pink tourmaline

Rose quartz

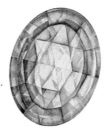

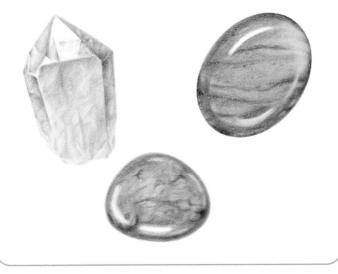

Throat Chakra

Considered the communication hub, this chakra is related to all aspects of physical communication and creative expression, especially conscious communication with intent. Self-expression, listening to and interacting with you are also associated with the throat chakra. Truth, clarity, knowledge and wisdom are all traits connected with the throat chakra. Cats don't always use their voice to communicate, so any actions related to their self-expression, such as conscious, deliberate inappropriate elimination, spiteful acts or actions based in jealousy or anger are all related to this chakra.

Location: Throat area.

Associated colour: Sky blue.

Associated glands/organs: Throat, thyroid, parathyroid, hypothalamus, mouth, teeth, vocal cords.

Possible imbalance: Depression, excessive or complete lack of vocalization, vocal issues, metabolism, hairballs, teething, thyroid issues, lack of discernment, knowledge used unwisely, attention-seeking and destructive behaviour, upper respiratory infection, coughing, inappropriate scratching, retaliation, dental issues, stomatitis (sore mouth), inflamed gums, tooth extractions, halitosis.

A balanced throat chakra can result in a cat who is communicative in a balanced and friendly way, interacts with you and others, is happy with her circumstances, is wise and is understanding of attention and devoted to others.

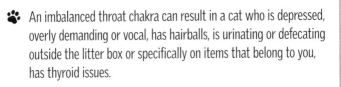 An imbalanced throat chakra can result in a cat who is depressed, overly demanding or vocal, has hairballs, is urinating or defecating outside the litter box or specifically on items that belong to you, has thyroid issues.

Spirit animal: The spirit or totem animal associated with the throat chakra is the bear. The bear relates to rhythm, flow, alignment and heeding our inner voice. Call in or ask bear energy to come forth to your feline companion to be with her for the purpose of healing her throat chakra.

Ways to stimulate the throat chakra: Play with your cat, communicate with her, sing to her, play music for her, meditate with her, and be creative around or with her.

Archangel: Michael is the archangel associated with the throat chakra. You can call upon Archangel Michael to balance your cat's energy related to the throat chakra, and at the same time to release any and all non-beneficial energies to be transmuted by the spiritual realm. Feel free to list any specifics you are aware of as you ask for assistance from the archangels.

Affirmations: You can create your own affirmation to suit your cat's particular situation or use one of the following:
"[Cat's name] communicates her wishes to me in acceptable ways."
"[Cat's name]'s vocalization habits are perfectly balanced."
"[Cat's name] has a cheerful demeanour."

Visualization: If you've determined that the throat chakra is imbalanced, first visualize it as it currently is, and then, on the count of three, visualize it coming into perfect balance. Then visualize "locking it in" to this balanced fashion so that it will stay balanced.

Colour therapy: Physically apply the colour sky blue to the throat chakra and rest of the body, as for the root chakra (see pages 56–7).

For crystal healing, pendulum dowsing and brain integration: Refer to these sections under the root chakra section (see pages 56–7).

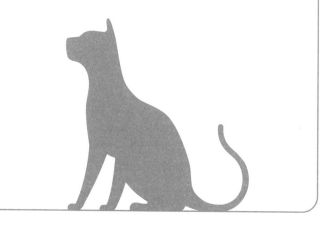

CRYSTALS THAT AID IN HEALING THE THROAT CHAKRA

Amazonite
Angelite
Aquamarine
Blue lace agate
Celestite
Lapis lazuli
Sodalite
Turquoise

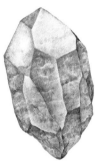

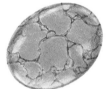

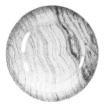

Sensing Chakra

Related to the sensory intake and transmission of sensory information to the brain. In other words, how our feline companions filter and assimilate all experiences that occur, and how they deal with any and all sensory stimuli (seeing, hearing, smelling, touching, feeling and even knowing). It is common for cats to be extra sensitive to sudden noises, unexpected occurrences they aren't prepared for or don't understand, and towards other cats and household companions; in fact, it's often their nature. But when this chakra is out of balance, even normally occurring circumstances can range from triggering to terrifying. Be sure to check and balance this chakra in any abandoned, feral or rescue cat. The sensing chakra is the reason cats have heightened sensing ability compared to humans.

Location: Bridge of the nose between the tip of the nose and the eyes.

Associated colour: Silver blue.

Associated glands/organs: Face, nose, eyes, ears, paw pads, whiskers, tail tip.

Possible imbalance: Over- or under-reacting to events, noises, circumstances or training cues; any imbalance of the eyes, ears, nose, tail, etc.; docked tails, clipped whiskers, blindness, deafness, inappropriate elimination, inappropriate scratching, aggression, intolerance, timidity, excessive licking, disliking nail trimming, eating plants and flowers.

- A balanced sensing chakra can result in a cat who is comfortable, confident, calm and trusting, and has a good awareness and perception of her senses, including seeing, hearing, smelling, touching and feeling.

- An imbalanced sensing chakra can result in a cat who is skittish, excitable, fearful, timid, dislikes having claws trimmed, lacking in her natural sensing and assimilation abilities; is an abandoned, feral or rescue cat.

Spirit animal: The spirit or totem animal associated with the sensing chakra is the turtle. The turtle relates to new opportunities, manifesting, awakening to and connecting with our primal senses. Call in or ask turtle energy to come forth to your feline companion to be with her for the purpose of healing her sensing chakra.

Ways to stimulate the sensing chakra: Meditate, stargaze or watch clouds with your cat; learn about and work with subtle energies from her; communicate with her.

Archangel: Metatron is the archangel associated with the sensing chakra. You can call upon Archangel Metatron to balance your cat's energy related to the sensing chakra, and at the same time to release any and all non-beneficial energies to be transmuted by the spiritual realm. Feel free to list any specifics you are aware of as you ask for assistance from the archangels.

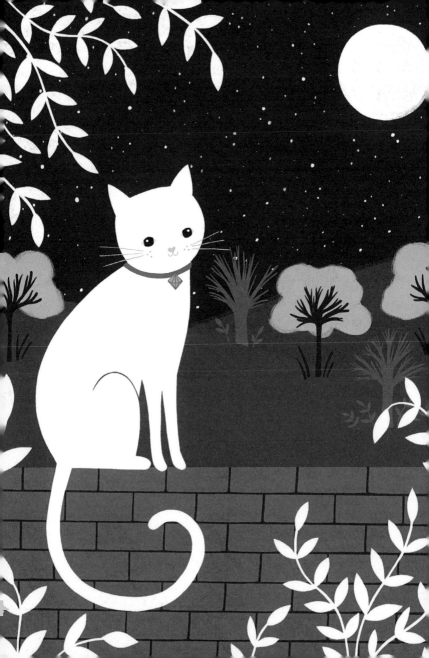

Affirmations: You can create your own affirmation to suit your cat's particular situation or use one of the following:

"[Cat's name] reacts calmly to normal day-to-day occurrences."

"[Cat's name] releases any and all tendencies to overreact."

"[Cat's name] is becoming more and more tolerant of other cats and household companions."

Visualization: If you've determined that the sensing chakra is imbalanced, first visualize it as it currently is, and then, on the count of three, visualize it coming into perfect balance. Then visualize "locking it in" to this balanced fashion so that it will stay balanced.

Colour therapy: Physically apply the colour silver blue to the sensing chakra and rest of the body, as for the root chakra (see pages 56–7).

For crystal healing, pendulum dowsing and brain integration: Refer to these sections under the root chakra section (see pages 56–7).

CRYSTALS THAT AID IN HEALING THE SENSING CHAKRA

Angelite	Chalcedony
Aquamarine	Lapis lazuli
Blue lace agate	Phantom quartz
Celestite	Sapphire

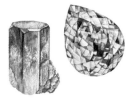

Third Eye Chakra
(Brow Chakra)

Related to psychic insight and universal connection. Self-acceptance, level-headedness, calmness, ability to focus, soul realization, concentration and devotion are important aspects of this chakra. It is another of the key areas for interspecies telepathic communication (also known as animal communication) with humans, as well as communication with others of their species and members of their household or clan. This chakra is very well developed in most animals, as they are easily in tune, aware and connected, unlike many humans. Also related to survival instinct, offering cats the focus and ability required to hunt for their food.

Location: Centre of the forehead above the eyes.

Associated colour: Indigo.

Associated glands/organs: Pituitary gland, pineal, ears, left eye, nose, fur, hair, skin.

Possible imbalance: Headaches, depression, boredom, concentration issues, hair loss, hearing loss, hyperactivity, post-traumatic pain or stress, allergies, skin allergies, over-grooming, feline acne, dandruff, hormone issues, nervous system, neurological issues, congestion, runny nose, allergies, ear issues including ear mites, eye issues including irritable eyes, conjunctivitis, cataracts.

A balanced third eye chakra can result in a cat who is accepting, calm, focused, aware, in tune, connected to her surroundings and others, connected psychically, a willing participant in interspecies telepathic communication.

 An imbalanced third eye chakra can result in a cat who is stressed, hyperactive, excitable, disconnected from her surroundings and others, uninterested in interspecies telepathic communication, experiences skin disorders or hair loss.

Spirit animal: The spirit or totem animal associated with the third eye chakra is the eagle. The eagle relates to vision, mysticism, power and healing. Call in or ask eagle energy to come forth to your feline companion to be with her for the purpose of healing her third eye chakra.

Ways to stimulate the third eye chakra: Meditate, stargaze or watch clouds with your cat, communicate with her, focus on bridging the gap between physical knowing and universal truth – conduct esoteric studies in the presence of your cat.

Archangel: Zadkiel is the archangel associated with the third eye chakra. You can call upon Archangel Zadkiel to balance your cat's energy related to the third eye chakra, and at the same time to release any and all non-beneficial energies to be transmuted by the spiritual realm. Feel free to list any specifics you are aware of as you ask for assistance from the archangels.

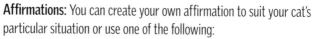

Affirmations: You can create your own affirmation to suit your cat's particular situation or use one of the following:

"[Cat's name] is calm and accepting."

"[Cat's name] enjoys communication with myself and others."

"[Cat's name] is at one with the Universe and her psychic connection."

Visualization: If you've determined that the third eye chakra is imbalanced, first visualize it as it currently is, and then, on the count of three, visualize it coming into perfect balance. Then visualize "locking it in" in this balanced fashion so that it will stay balanced.

Colour therapy: Physically apply the colour indigo to the third eye chakra and rest of the body, as for the root chakra (see pages 56–7).

For crystal healing, pendulum dowsing and brain integration: Refer to these sections under the root chakra section (see pages 56–7).

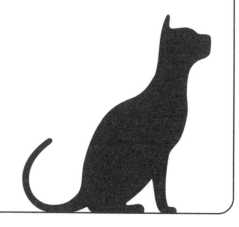

CRYSTALS THAT AID IN HEALING THE THIRD EYE CHAKRA

Azurite

Chalcedony

Iolite

Lapiz lazuli

Moonstone

Opal

Pearl

Selenite

Soadalite

Star sapphire

Suglite

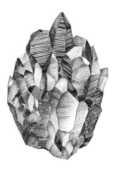

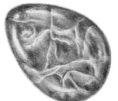

Crown Chakra

Related to the life force connection with the infinite (with God/Goddess, the Universe, spirit). Think of this as the centre responsible for the soul (or essence) of your cat, inhabiting her body. It governs a cat's connection with the world around her and provides access to the vast collective consciousness and universal wisdom, enabling the ability to communicate naturally on subjects far greater than might be expected. This is the chakra of divine wisdom, deep understanding, connection with the world around her, selfless service and perception beyond space and time; exactly what you'd hope for from your cat.

Location: Top of the head.

Associated colours: Violet or white.

Associated glands/organs: Cerebral cortex, skull, brain, central nervous system, right eye, pineal gland.

Possible imbalance: Neurological issues, grief, depression, disorientation, fear, headaches, hyperactive, panic attacks, boredom, pining, senility, separation anxiety, stress, tension, sleep issues, training issues, perception of reality, eye issues including irritable eyes, conjunctivitis, cataracts.

🐾 A balanced crown chakra can result in a cat who is relaxed and well-integrated in her body on this earthly plane; well-connected

to source energy, the spiritual realm and the world around her;
able to tap into universal wisdom, aware of and connected to her
mission; strong self-healing ability and ability to heal in general.

🐾 An imbalanced crown chakra can result in a cat who suffers
the injustices done to her species as a whole, individually as
well as through world events and natural disasters; experiences
headaches, anxiety, pain, and neurological issues.

Spirit animal: The spirit or totem animal associated with the crown
chakra is the bee. The bee relates to new choices, fertility, fulfilment
and spiritual guidance. Call in or ask bee energy to come forth to
your feline companion to be with her for the purpose of healing her
crown chakra.

Ways to stimulate the crown chakra: Focus on mutual dreams and
intentions; connect to the spirit and practise metaphysical studies in
the presence of your cat; connect to your mission in the presence of
your cat; focus on bridging the gap between physical knowing and
universal truth.

Archangel: Gabriel is the archangel associated with the crown
chakra. You can call upon Archangel Gabriel to balance your cat's
energy related to the crown chakra, and at the same time to release
any and all non-beneficial energies to be transmuted by the spiritual
realm. Feel free to list any specifics you are aware of as you ask for
assistance from the archangels.

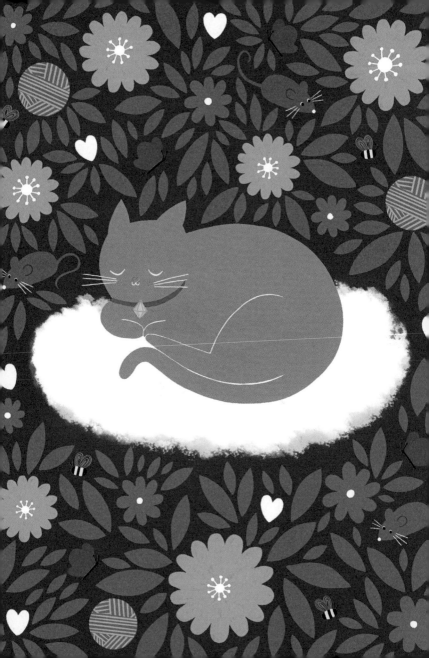

Affirmations: You can create your own affirmation to suit your cat's particular situation or use one of the following:
"[Cat's name] is comfortable in her skin."
"[Cat's name]'s brain and neurological system are fully balanced."
"[Cat's name] has complete access to the collective consciousness and universal wisdom."

Visualization: If you've determined that the crown chakra is imbalanced, first visualize it as it currently is, and then, on the count of three, visualize it coming into perfect balance. Then visualize "locking it in" to this balanced fashion so that it will stay balanced.

Colour therapy: Physically apply the colour violet to the crown chakra and rest of the body, as for the root chakra (see pages 56–7).

For crystal healing, pendulum dowsing and brain integration: Refer to these sections under the root chakra section (see pages 56–7).

CRYSTALS THAT AID IN HEALING THE CROWN CHAKRA

Amethyst	Lepidolite
Diamond	Purple fluorite
Herkimer diamond	Quartz
Lemurian diamond	Violet tourmaline

Brachial Chakra

A very powerful major energy centre in cats relating to connection, transformation and energy flow. This chakra is a central hub from which you can access all the other chakras, both major and minor, as well as gleaning an entire picture of what is going on in the energy field of your cat. It is another key chakra where cats and their humans can connect, bond and communicate, and a great chakra to work with to re-establish a weak or lost connection with one another. It is a place from which you can treat the whole body and entire chakra system, and it is recommended as the starting point for any hands-on healing work.

Location: Either side of the lower neck, just in front of the shoulder blade, accessing the brachial plexus nerves.

Associated colour: Black.

Associated glands/organs: Heart, thymus, lungs, respiratory system, circulatory system, chest, front legs and paws.

Possible imbalance: A cat with a brachial chakra that needs balancing can experience almost any imbalance conceivable, especially those related to the head, neck and front portion of the body; a cat with cancer; a cat who dislikes human touch or being picked up. Be sure to balance this chakra for any cat being introduced to a new home as well as abandoned, rescue or feral cats.

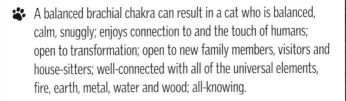

- A balanced brachial chakra can result in a cat who is balanced, calm, snuggly; enjoys connection to and the touch of humans; open to transformation; open to new family members, visitors and house-sitters; well-connected with all of the universal elements, fire, earth, metal, water and wood; all-knowing.

- An imbalanced brachial chakra can result in a cat who has imbalanced energy in any area, but especially the head, neck and front legs; is disconnected emotionally; nervous; dislikes human touch and any kind of deeper connection.

Spirit animal: The spirit or totem animal associated with the brachial chakra is the raven. The raven relates to the circle of life, illumination, magic and mysticism. Ask raven energy to come forth to your feline companion to be with her for the purpose of healing her brachial chakra.

Ways to stimulate the brachial chakra: Any and all of the ways mentioned for the other major chakras, depending on the issue; focusing particularly on deepening your connection with and interspecies telepathic communication with your cat.

Archangel: All of the archangels (Uriel, Chamuel, Jophiel, Raphael, Michael, Metatron, Zadkiel and Gabriel) are associated with the brachial chakra. Call upon any of them to balance your cat's brachial chakra, and at the same time to release any and all non-beneficial energies. Feel free to list any specifics you are aware of as you ask for assistance from the archangels.

Affirmations: You can create your own affirmation to suit your cat's particular situation or use one of the following:
"[Cat's name]'s energy flows perfectly and harmoniously."
"[Cat's name] easily bonds with myself and other family members."
"[Cat's name] enjoys physical touch."

Visualization: If you've determined that the brachial chakra is imbalanced, first visualize it as it currently is, and then, on the count of three, visualize it coming into perfect balance. Then visualize "locking it in" to this balanced fashion so that it will stay balanced.

Colour therapy: Physically apply the colour black to the brachial chakra and rest of the body, as for the root chakra (see pages 56–7).

For crystal healing, pendulum dowsing and brain integration: Refer to these sections under the root chakra section (see pages 56–7).

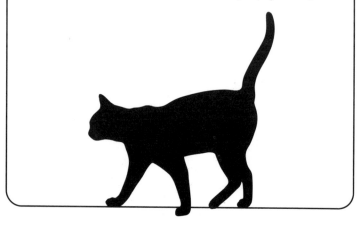

CRYSTALS THAT AID IN HEALING THE BRACHIAL CHAKRA

Black onyx

Black pearl

Black tourmaline

Boji stone

Jet

Shungite

Snowflake obsidian

Tiger eye

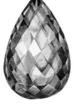

As well as any of the crystals listed to aid in the healing of any of the other major chakras.

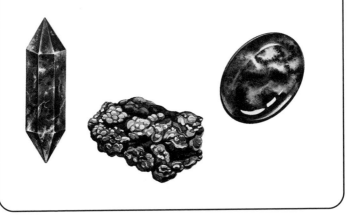

THE MINOR CHAKRAS

Your cat's minor chakras govern and relate to very specific aspects of one or more of her major chakras. It can be advantageous to work with the minor chakras when you are concerned with a very specific or specialized sub-issue of a major chakra, as the minor chakras allow us to direct and clear energies specifically related to that issue. For example, the body language chakra is just one aspect of the throat chakra, and when working on the body language chakra, you are directing energy in a more specialized fashion (or direction). In many cases, working on the associated major chakra will handle all your cat's needs, but I wanted to provide options as well as leaving it up to the higher self of your cat to determine which is in her highest and best interest.

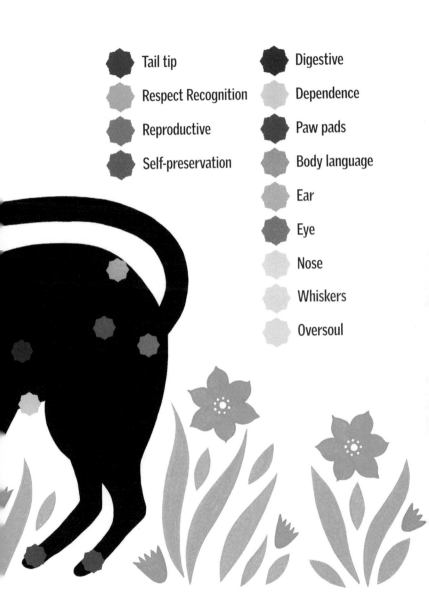

Tail tip

Respect Recognition

Reproductive

Self-preservation

Digestive

Dependence

Paw pads

Body language

Ear

Eye

Nose

Whiskers

Oversoul

Self-preservation Chakra

Sub-chakra of the root chakra; see the root chakra for further details (see pages 54–7).

The self-preservation chakra governs the energy that runs down the hind legs of the cat. It is known as the fight-or-flight, adrenal or red-alert state chakra. Its state is representative of the stress or energy drain in cats living in unharmonious or less-than-ideal circumstances. This chakra is frequently out of balance in rescue, feral and abused cats. It is also an issue for cats living in situations with others (cats, dogs or humans) that they don't tolerate or get along with.

Location: Hip joint.

Associated colour: Red.

Possible imbalance: Aggression, dominance, bullying, territoriality, intolerance, submissiveness, inappropriate urination or defecation, hip dysplasia, arthritis, abuse, fear, anxiety.

Reproductive Chakra

Sub-chakra of the root and sexual progression chakras; see the root chakra (pages 54–7) and sexual progression chakra (pages 58–61) for further details.

The reproductive chakra governs all aspects of reproduction including heat cycles, natural mating instinct, drive to propagate the species, hormone imbalances, false pregnancies and mammary gland issues.

Location: Reproductive organs.

Associated colour: Red-orange.

Possible imbalance: False pregnancy, breeding issues of all sorts, irregular heat cycles, ovarian cysts, spay/neuter issues, maternal instinct.

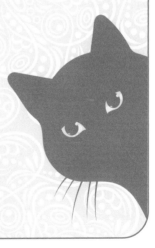

Digestive Chakra

Sub-chakra of the solar plexus chakra; see the solar plexus chakra for further details (see pages 62–5).

Governs all aspects of digestion, including eating and weight issues, hunting abilities and the natural instinct to avoid poisons and other inedibles.

Location: Tip of the liver.

Associated colour: Rust red.

Possible imbalance: Vomiting, diarrhoea, stomach upset, colitis, acid reflux, scavenging, anorexia, ravenous appetite, or a foreign object in the digestive system.

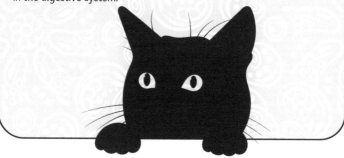

Respect Recognition Chakra

Sub-chakra of the sexual progression chakra; see the sexual progression chakra for further details (see pages 58–61).

Governs territory and social customs beyond the cat's household and family members. Also known as the friend or foe centre.

Location: Spine above internal reproductive organs.

Associated colour: Gold.

Possible imbalance: Over-protective, over-concerned, or over-responsible cats, territorial issues, poor breeding issues (in nature the best genes are deferred to, to propagate a species) and any other issues related to procreation.

Dependence Chakra

Sub-chakra of the solar plexus chakra; see the solar plexus chakra for further details (see pages 62–5).

The place of independence, trust and obedience with people, and of dominance or submission with other animals.

Location: Underbelly below gallbladder.

Associated colour: Citron yellow.

Possible imbalance: Insecurity, trust issues, training issues, dominance, submissiveness, nervousness and fear.

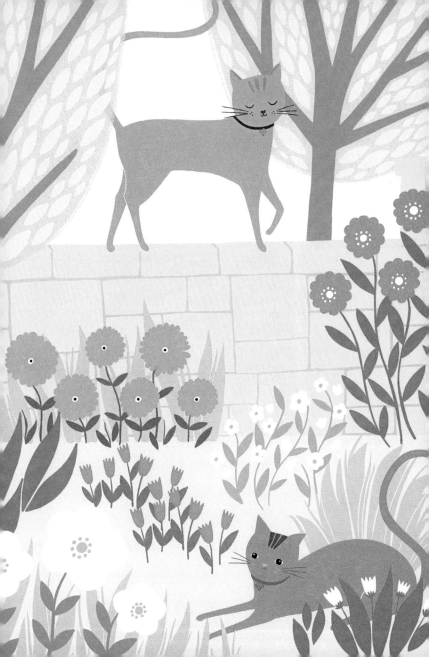

Body Language Chakra

Sub-chakra of the throat chakra; see the throat chakra for further details (see pages 70–3).

Governs behaviour in intentional communication (tail wagging, purring, pawing, smiling, imitating humans). Controls the energy that runs along the spine, down the legs and into the paws.

Location: Behind the throat chakra.

Associated colour: Blue.

Possible imbalance: Excessive vocalization or communication, lack of vocalization or communication, any kind of intentional physical communication, such as pawing and other behaviours.

Eye Chakra

Sub-chakra of the sensing chakra; see the sensing chakra for further details (see pages 74–7).

Associated with the sensing chakra and related to any issues pertaining to the eyes and vision.

Location: Eyes.

Associated colour: Violet or lavender.

Possible imbalance: Cataracts, glaucoma, blindness, fading vision, runny eyes, eyelash issues, eye infections and allergies.

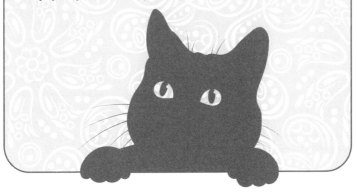

Ear Chakra

Sub-chakra of the sensing chakra; see the sensing chakra for further details (see pages 74–7).

Associated with the sensing chakra and related to any issues pertaining to the ears and hearing.

Location: Base of the ears.

Associated colours: Aqua or blue.

Possible imbalance: Ear infections, hearing issues, deafness, ear mites, rhinitis and allergies.

Nose Chakra

Sub-chakra of the sensing chakra; see the sensing chakra for further details (see pages 74–7).

Associated with the sensing chakra and related to any issues pertaining to the nose and sense of smell (a cat's sense of smell is said to be 14 times greater than a human's).

Location: Tip of the nose.

Associated colour: Silver blue.

Possible imbalance: Allergies, sinus infections, sensitivity, lack of smell, picky eater, respiratory issues.

Whiskers Chakra

Sub-chakra of the sensing chakra; see the sensing chakra for further details (see pages 74–7).

Associated with the sensing chakra and related to any issues pertaining to the whiskers.

Location: Face beside the mouth.

Associated colour: Silver blue.

Possible imbalance: Infection, whisker fatigue, clipped or missing whiskers due to injury, issues related to face, mouth, teeth, gums and tongue.

Paw Pads Chakra

Sub-chakra of the sensing chakra; see the sensing chakra for further details (see pages 74–7).

Associated with the sensing chakra and related to any issues pertaining to the paw pads.

Location: Bottom of the feet.

Associated colour: Ruby red.

Possible imbalance: Amputations, nail clipping concerns, any other issues of the paw pads.

Tail Tip Chakra

Sub-chakra of the sensing and root chakras; see the sensing chakra (pages 74–7) and the root chakra (pages 54–7) for further details.

Associated with the sensing and root chakras and related to any issues pertaining to the tip of the tail.

Location: Tip of the tail (if the tail has been cropped, it is where the tail would have ended).

Associated colour: Dark red.

Possible imbalance: Docked tails, amputations, bite wounds, abrasions, infections and any other tail issues.

Oversoul Chakra
(Transpersonal Point Chakra)

Sub-chakra of the third eye and crown chakras; see the third eye chakra (pages 78–81) and the crown chakra (pages 82–5) for further details.

The connection of an individual cat to their higher self, spirit and the Universe, as well as their connection to their soul group; also known as an oversoul.

Location: Base of the skull or above the crown chakra.

Associated colours: White or silver.

Possible imbalance: Any imbalance related to the third eye or crown chakra, especially those connected with the unseen realms, telepathy and psychic insight. With this chakra, I usually wait until it comes up to be balanced and just trust that it is in divine order.

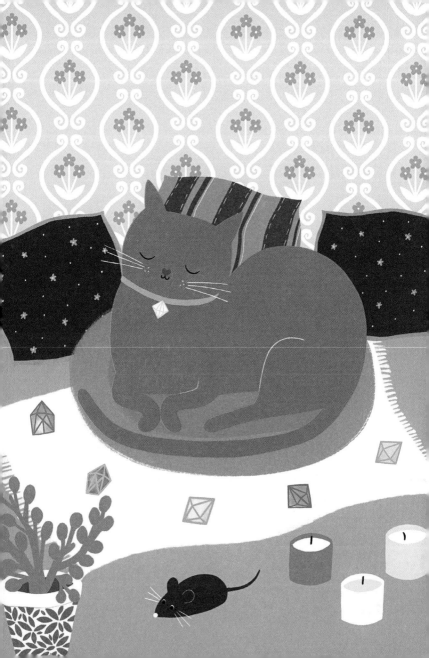

PART THREE
WHOLE-BODY HEALING

The tools and techniques featured in this section work with the body as an integrated whole to facilitate healing in the energy field and therefore the chakras. They include crystal healing, the use of flower essences and gem elixirs, and how to use a pendulum for dowsing.

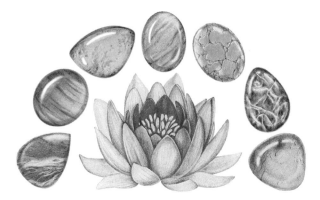

CRYSTAL HEALING

This technique uses crystals and other stones to heal, balance and protect. Crystals encourage positive, healing energy to flow into the body and displace negative, harmful energy.

What Are Crystals?

Crystals and gemstones are enchanted gifts from the Earth that can promote extraordinary healing in the energy field as well as in the chakras – in both humans and animals. Since felines possess a natural receptivity, crystals work well to draw to themselves the precise energies they require to heal. Crystals are formed naturally in the Earth, and the term "crystal" refers to any precious gem, mineral, stone, fossil or resin that has a measurable charge and produces an electrical pulse.

Important Notes

🐾 It is my preference (and your cat's), especially when working with sensitive animals, that your crystal healing work be set up in such a way that they be allowed to come and go from the crystal energy and not have it forced upon them at all times.

🐾 Certain crystals, including malachite, cinnabar and peacock ore, are toxic. *Avoid using these stones with cats.*

🐾 Always make sure the crystals you use are large enough not to be ingested by any animal or small child in the household.

🐾 Crystal healing is not meant to replace veterinary care.

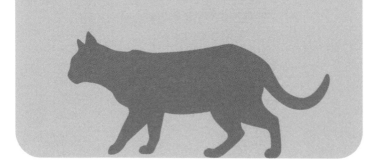

How Crystal Healing Works

Each crystal has a specific vibrational frequency and amplitude, which reverberates or resonates with and attracts the energies of certain qualities or traits to your cat. Crystal healing is a non-invasive healing technique that works on all levels of consciousness: physical, emotional, mental and spiritual.

Clearing crystals
Before you begin using crystals with your cat, it is important to clear the energy of the crystal. This can be done by leaving the crystal out in the sunlight or moonlight, with smoke from a smudge stick, or with your intention.

Programming crystals
A crystal can be programmed for a specific use simply by placing it in your hand. Then, while you are in a healing state, assign it a particular job or task; ask it to help a particular animal with a particular situation or issue. This can be done by saying the words either out loud, or silently, inside your head.

For example, hold a piece of blue lace agate (a cooling stone) in your hand and ask it to help calm your cat's excessive vocalization and demanding nature. Then place it in your cat's environment and watch it work.

Ways to Work with Crystals and Your Cat

Place some crystals in her space. Affix a crystal pendant onto your cat's collar (if she wears one), zip a crystal into her bedding or place one under her favourite chair.

🐾

Give your cat a crystal massage. Massage her with a crystal wand or other smooth, tumbled stone. This can be done either on the body or in the aura.

🐾

Place a crystal in her water bowl (make sure it is large enough not to be ingested by any animal in the household). This will infuse her water (and thus her) with the properties of the crystal.

🐾

Create a crystal layout, spread around a stationary animal or at a favourite sunning spot where your cat loves to nap.

🐾

Send the frequency of a particular healing crystal to your cat (similar to the technique you learned in Part Two when sending colour to the chakra).

Use this statement: "[Cat's name], receive [name of crystal] perfectly now, on all levels, all dimensions, all aspects known and unknown, now and for all time."

❖

Wear crystals yourself as jewellery when you are around your feline friend.

❖

Protect her space. This can be done by placing four crystal points in the corner of a crate, cat bed or your feline companion's favourite part of the house, with the intention that they are for protection. Clear quartz is most commonly used for this purpose.

❖

Crystals can be used intentionally to add or remove energy from your cat or kitten. It's beneficial to add energy to a weak cat or kitten who is not thriving, but in the case of an animal with a lot of heat and inflammation present, such as an elderly cat with arthritis, removing energy will serve her better.

Increasing and Decreasing Energy

To send energy into an area:

🐾 Hold a clear quartz crystal with a point on one end, 6–12 in (15–30 cm) away from your cat, with the point towards the problem area.

🐾 Then circle clockwise as you move the crystal closer and closer to the area you are treating while setting the intention to add energy and vitality.

To remove energy from an area, do the exact opposite:

🐾 Hold a clear quartz crystal with a point on one end, 1 in (2.5 cm) or so away from your cat, with the tip pointing away from the problem area (but not directly at you).

🐾 Then circle counterclockwise as you move the crystal further and further away from the area you are treating while setting the intention to add energy and vitality.

🐾 You can place the pointed end of a crystal on each side of a problem area and ask the crystal to increase the energy in an area or to clear an energy blockage. Don't rely on this if your cat has eaten a foreign object; it only works for energy blockages.

The Four Master Healers

There are four master healer crystals that can be used for any and all conditions, at any point on the body: clear quartz, rose quartz, amethyst and smoky quartz. These are great crystals to have in your collection.

Let's look at some of the other crystals that can be used for a variety of feline issues. Once you've familiarized yourself with crystal work, you can find the crystals that resonate specifically with your cat's issues in the box below.

Crystals for Cats

Amber: Dispels negative energy. Detoxifying, purifying and protective. Good for digestive problems.

Amethyst: Soothes fears and stresses; calms an anxious cat.

Aventurine: Heals emotional scars and promotes confidence.

Blue lace agate: Anti-inflammatory and cooling. Good for demanding, vocal, or hungry cats.

Boji stone: Tissue regeneration, strengthens the meridians, and enhances partnership and cooperation. Can be used to help with training issues.

Carnelian: Builds confidence and concentration, and helps to increase the appetite. Strengthens the vital life force and increases the will to live.

Citrine: Good for emotional, sensory overload. Boosts the immune system. Any of the yellow stones can be used for issues of the bladder, urinary tract, and kidneys.

Copper: Can be used for purification or arthritic conditions, as in for humans.

Covellite: Can be used for any serious illness requiring detoxification.

Fluorite: A fabulous gait balancer. A detoxifier that helps improve the mental focus and assimilation of food.

Hematite: Good for emotional boundaries. It can also be used for any issues related to the blood or bleeding.

Jet: A resin used as a protective talisman since the Stone Age. Grounding and useful in the breaking of negative patterns.

Lapis lazuli: Can be used for respiratory issues, detoxifying, enhancing the energy flow, and to boost the energy.

Moonstone: Calming, can be used for any female-related procreation situation or issue in your feline.

Rose quartz: The crystal of joy and unconditional love. Good for animals that are abused, abandoned, or neglected. It's also good for cats that have to tolerate something they'd rather not. This is one of my favourite go-to crystals.

Selenite: Clears energy blocks; promotes peace and calming. One of the best crystals for help in the treatment of any type of cancer.

Smoky quartz: Grounds, calms, releases stress and nervousness. One of my favourite go-to crystals.

Turquoise: A great healer stone that can also be used for protection, tissue regeneration, or as a systemic tonic.

FLOWER ESSENCES AND GEM ELIXIRS

Both flower essences and gem elixirs contain the energy of the plant or stone from which they are derived. These can then be used to bring forth positive effects or treat particular issues.

What Is a Flower Essence?

All living beings have a consciousness, and that also includes flowers. For nearly a century, flower essences have provided powerful, vibrational energy that heals humans and animals alike.

The specific life-force pattern of the flower is contained in its vibrational frequency, and this is the purpose behind creating flower essences. The vibrational and energetic frequencies of the flower are captured in spring water and preserved, often with a type of pure alcohol like vodka. When the essence is applied topically or taken internally, it awakens certain qualities in the human or animal taking it, drawing forth desired traits or positive attributes and encouraging emotional balance.

The history of flower essences

Flower essences were developed in England in the 1930s by Dr Edward Bach, a physician and researcher who set out to harness the power of flowers for healing and wellbeing. Bach Flower Remedies were originally developed for humans, but they have since been found to be incredibly helpful for animals as well – especially since animals' energy systems are less complicated. Cats are closer to flowers, both physically and energetically, and thus they respond well to flower essences. Through the process of absorbing and embodying the vibrational frequency of the flower, your cat can heal physically, emotionally and mentally, in a number of ways.

Since flower essences are completely fragrance-free and non-toxic, they are perfectly safe and ideal to use with your cat. Unlike essential oils, with which they are often confused and contain chemical constituents that can be toxic to cats, flower essences are completely safe and have no known side effects. Flower essences won't interfere with medications, so they integrate easily with both holistic and allopathic medicines.

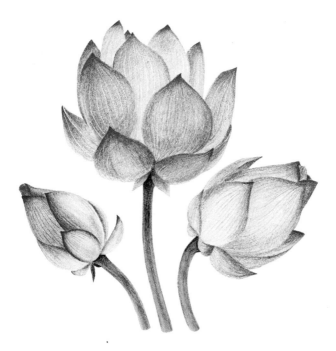

What Is a Gem Elixir?

A gem elixir is made in a very similar way to a flower essence. Instead of a flower, a crystal is chosen and soaked in spring water to capture the vibrational frequency of the crystal in the water. Just as with flowers, different crystals offer different frequencies, energies and benefits through the gem elixir. Also, gem elixirs are equally safe and beneficial to both people and animals.

How to Select Flower Essences and Gem Elixirs

When choosing gem elixirs and flower essences, it's helpful to note that both have no harmful effect on those who do not need them. Indeed, it is recommended that all animals and humans in the household take the same group of essences to integrate and balance all of the energies and produce an environment of harmony. Very often, our animal companions are absorbing energies and emotions from the people in their family, so this can help to clear up any sources of their imbalance.

With this in mind, you can use methods such as dowsing or muscle testing to match the essence to the person and/or cat energetically. I have found these to be the best methods, but there are others that work just as well. You can choose a flower essence for yourself and your cat by determining which flower you are strongly drawn to, or you can

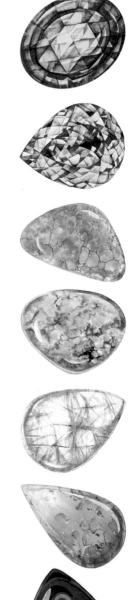

also look at your cat's personality and temperament and find an essence that matches based on the essence description (you can look this up online or in books, charts, etc.; we will talk more about this later). Focus on the traits you'd like your cat to release – traits like rigidity or persistence – as well as the positive ones you'd like to restore or strengthen.

When selecting flower essences, you can pick as many as five or six at a time. As mentioned earlier, it is not harmful to select the wrong remedy; if one is not needed, it won't cause your cat any ill effects. However, too many remedies at once will be less effective than fewer well-chosen ones, so try to tune in to your inner self and follow where it leads for you and your cat. Then, trust your cat to let you know what is and isn't working for her.

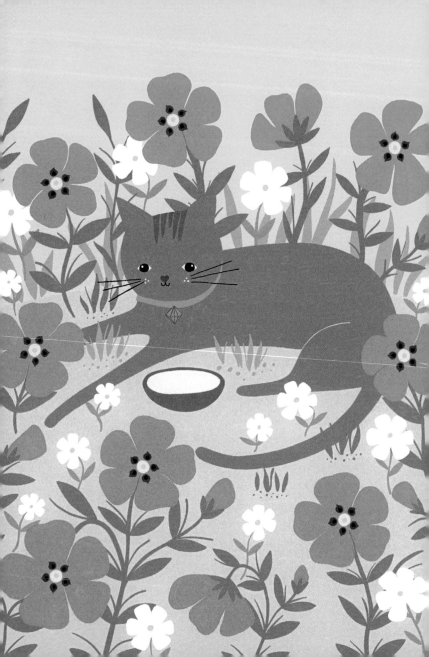

Ways to Administer Flower Essences and Gem Elixirs

The best way to administer flower essences is in your cat's water. Add two to four drops of the essence to each bowl of water. Having multiple cats (and other animal companions) sharing one water bowl is fine. For humans, since it's recommended that we take the same essences as our feline friends, a few drops may be put directly under the tongue or in a glass of water and sipped at least four times per day – more often is even better.

For ease of dispensing a number of flower essences at one time, you can make what's known as a stock bottle, which is a blend of various essences in a clean 1-oz (25-ml) glass bottle with a dropper. You can do this by adding 10 to 20 drops of each essence and filling it the rest of the way with spring water. Squirt a dropperful into your cat's mouth four times a day (with a plastic dropper for safety if using with cats) or empty the dropper into her water bowl as described above. Stock bottles must be kept in the refrigerator and will last up to 30 days without contamination. Please note that most cats strongly dislike having the essences squirted into their mouths and it's best to respect their wishes, as adding additional stress will defeat the objective of the healing process (or goal).

Flower essences can also be applied topically on your cat – preferably in a spot where there is no fur, such as on the paw pads, around the muzzle or on the ears. The shoulders or back (part the hair first) are often the easiest. This is particularly recommended for cats that don't drink frequently enough to ingest the essences four times per day.

As each flower essence or gem elixir has its own unique energy, it is very important to approach giving your cat flower essences or gem elixirs with a positive intention and prayerful ritual when offering them to her. Be decisive and intentional on how you want them to help your animal companion with their healing, respecting the nature spirits involved and the healing power of the essences, and say your prayer or declaration that it will be so.

How to Use Flower Essences and Gem Elixirs in Chakra Healing

When you have a specific trait or behaviour that you're trying to heal in your cat's chakras, it can be useful to own a flower essence guide or pamphlet. For example, if your cat exhibits fear, which is associated with the root chakra, you can look up "fear" in your guide and find out which essence addresses it. If you look up the Bach Flower Remedies, you will see that mimulus, aspen and rock rose are the ideal remedies for fear. You can read about each of the essences and decide whether you feel it's best to give your cat just one or two, or all three together.

TIP: Always store flower essences in a cool, dry place away from sunlight and harmful frequencies like the microwave, as they may have a negative effect on them.

If your cat has been rescued, there's a good chance she has several traits that need healing, such as fear (as previously mentioned); feeling overwhelmed, discouraged or hopeless; shock or trauma. These traits can have an impact on several of your cat's chakras. If you look up the Bach Flower Remedies for these traits, you will see that as well as the essences for fear mentioned above, their remedies are elm, gentian, gorse and star of Bethlehem.

Then, you can give your cat the four essences mentioned above, plus one or two of the remedies for fear mentioned initially. You can give these to her all together, or another option would be to choose the ones that seem to be needed the most at the time based on the descriptions in your guide. You can give your cat those for at least four weeks, and then once you've seen some benefit, switch and give her the rest of them.

These are just a few examples of ways you can administer flower essences or gem elixirs – use your intuition and take guidance from your cat. Be ready to listen for clues on how she's responding. Keep in mind that there are many makers of flower essences and gem elixirs with numerous remedies in their catalogues. Therefore, there are far too many to list here; I suggest doing some research and finding one that works for you and your cat on your healing journey together.

PENDULUM DOWSING

Also known as questing or divining, dowsing can be done with a pendulum, a couple of other lesser-known devices, or in the case of an advanced dowser, it can be done without any equipment. A technique used since ancient times, dowsing is a wonderful way to tap into your intuition, heal and deepen the bond with your feline companion. It can also be used to communicate with your cat and to help find her if she gets lost. Everything, it seems, can be affected in a positive way with your good intention and a dowsing system.

Your specific questions, the language used and even your thoughts are very important to dowsing, and your results will be in direct proportion to how well you ask questions and manage your thoughts and how strongly you intend to emit and radiate healing.

Dowsing System

A dowsing system is simply the name given to any type of organized system of dowsing, which contains certain conditions, predetermined by you. You may ask your dowsing system to do specific things for you, such as clear a specific energy or release a particular emotion or pattern.

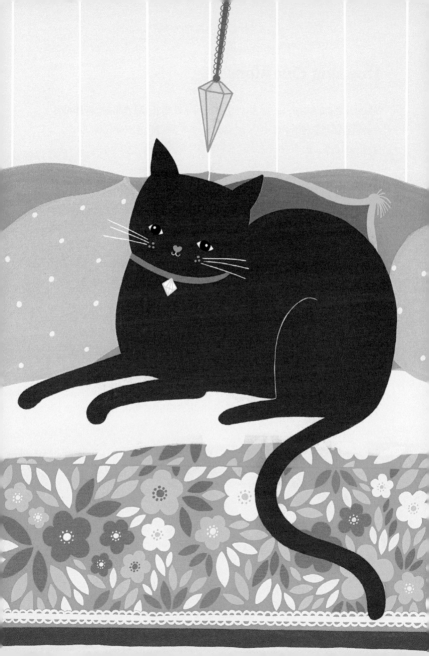

Dowsing Questions

Your dowsing is only as good as the questions that you ask; all questions must be as clear as possible and have a "yes" or "no" answer; the more specific they are, including time frame, the better.

- A good dowsing question is, "Is it in Tiger's highest and best good to trim his nails today?"

- A not-so-good dowsing question is, "Should I trim Tiger's nails?" This question doesn't address when or in whose best interest it is.

Intention

Your intention is everything in dowsing, so always be sure and very clear about it. Do your best to still your mind and let go of any preconceived judgements, biases, fears or expectations so that you can maintain complete neutrality. Ask only for the "light of truth" to come forth and intend that all dowsing sessions conducted come from an energy of love.

Brain Waves and Dowsing

When we are in a "dowsing state", our brain waves are measurably different from when we are awake, sleeping or meditating.

Preparing Yourself to Dowse

Readying ourselves energetically for dowsing is as important as the actual dowsing itself, as our accuracy as dowsers is completely dependent on us being balanced, centred, grounded, hydrated and focused. If your dowsing is off at all, I recommend that you come back to these basic preparatory steps. Even advanced dowsers are encouraged to follow them.

Tips for Effective Dowsing

Make sure you are grounded: Grounding, which you learned about in Part One, is being connected to Mother Earth and integrated in your physical body.

Quiet the mind: Bring yourself to a calm, meditative state, releasing all the cares and concerns of the day.

Protect yourself (and your pendulum): Bubble yourself in white light and/or say a protection statement or prayer.

Be hydrated: Always be well hydrated with water when doing pendulum work.

Call in your healing team: You learned about your healing team in Part One.

How to Dowse

 Hold the pendulum string or chain between your thumb and index finger approximately 2–3 in (5–7.5 cm) up from the pendulum. Gather up the rest of the string or chain into your hand; do not allow it to dangle down. Some beginners find it easier to hold the pendulum with a longer string, and you can do this, but it will take longer for the answers to show themselves through the pendulum swing.

 Start moving the pendulum in a neutral, to-and-fro swing. From this place, ask your pendulum for a "yes". Then ask for a "no". Make a note of what you get.

Basic Dowsing

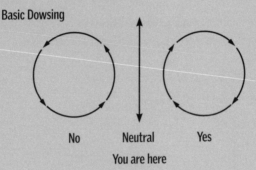

No   Neutral   Yes
You are here

 Be aware that if you're holding the pendulum over a specific body part and are not being specific in the question you are asking, you may be receiving the polarity (or spin) of that part of the body, so it is best to ask with your pendulum away from body parts (yours or your animal's) and be very clear in what you're asking.

 When the pendulum gives you your answer, stop asking your question and trust it.

It's All About Energy

The answer you get from your pendulum is simply the effect of neuromuscular changes in your hands as a result of your body's reaction to the answer to the question asked. We are able to receive this information, as we are all part of the collective consciousness or universal energy and therefore have access to all of the answers of the Universe.

When you ask a question in dowsing, you are tapping into that energy, and your body is receiving the answer. The pendulum is just a tool to help your mind see what your body is feeling (or already knows on some level). When asking questions in dowsing, they must be very clear and concise and must require only a "yes" or "no" answer. All dowsing must be for the highest and best good of all concerned, and it must come from a place of love and light.

Dowsing will not work if you are using it for personal gain, to infringe on another's privacy or to cause evil or hardship for another.

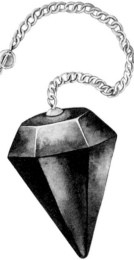

When facilitating healings for another, we are also healing ourselves.

Working on Your Cat: Starting a Session

Use this procedure to start and conduct a session.

Ask for permission
Start by asking for your cat's higher-self permission to work on her. Ask if it's in the highest and best good for both you and her (these are two separate questions).

Connecting energy fields
See diagram and exercise in Part One (pages 10–19).

Determine the issue
Determine the issue you wish to address and your intention for the session. Remember that the sky is the limit. Dowsing can be done for physical, emotional, mental and spiritual issues – basically, anything you can think of. For example, your goal for a session might be: to eliminate spraying, to increase peace and harmony, to ease your cat's nerves during a visit to the veterinarian, or to help align her energies to a difficult housemate. Please note that more than one issue can be worked on in a typical dowsing session.

Programming your pendulum for "yes" and "no"

Say, "Give me a yes", and wait for your pendulum to give it to you. Then, do the same for "no".

I recommend programming your pendulum to circle to the right for "yes", and to the left for "no", if it doesn't already do so. To do this, simply spin it to the right intentionally and say, "This is yes", and hold it in that spin for 60 seconds, and then spin it intentionally to the left and say, "This is no", and hold it in that spin for 60 seconds. After each answer, always bring your pendulum manually back to a neutral swinging position, to and fro.

Then check your "yes" and "no" again.

Dowsing for a priority item

When we are checking for an item (or chakra) that requires healing or balancing, it is in the best interest of our cat if we ask for the "priority". This means that if there are three chakras to be balanced in a session, or two crystal frequencies to be sent, that we be shown the one that is most important to do first. This is because sometimes when one item is balanced or cleared, it naturally takes care of some of the others, so when asking for and working by priority, we are maximizing the benefit of our healing.

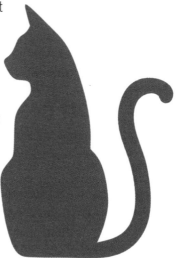

Working on Your Cat: Ending a Session

Use this procedure to end a session.

Ask if it's complete
Ask if everything that needs to be cleared or balanced at the moment is complete (as much as you understand and your cat is ready for at this time). Always have the intention that you will balance, heal or clear (by priority) as much as is appropriate in the time you have available.

Lock in your work
Use the following statement:

"[Cat's name], receive these healing energies with the love that is intended. Lock it into every cell, every fibre and every level of your being, in all dimensions, now and for all time."

Exercise: Disconnecting energy fields exercise
This is described in Part One (see steps 10–11 on page 15).

Sending a Frequency

Use the following statement when sending the frequency of a colour, crystal, flower essence or gem elixir to your cat:

"[Cat's name], receive [frequency being sent] perfectly now on all levels, all dimensions, all aspects, known and unknown, now and for all time."

Checking Your Cat's Chakras with Dowsing

There are a number of ways to check your cat's chakras (or your own) with dowsing.

 You may dowse over each of their chakras just above their physical body and ask to be shown the spin of each chakra (which is simply the energy flow). From there, you can ask that the chakra come into perfect balance as you are swinging your pendulum to and fro, in neutral. Then, after a short time, say 10 to 20 seconds, ask if it is fully balanced.

 Conversely, you can go chakra by chakra, asking one by one if each of them needs balancing right now. You would do this with your pendulum in your dominant hand and while touching the area of each chakra on your cat, or in your cat's aura with your non-dominant hand.

 You can simply make a list (handwritten or typed) of the cat chakras and dowse through them, using a pointer in your non-dominant, non-dowsing hand, and asking one by one if each chakra needs balancing.

 You may dowse the chakra charts shown in Part Two (see pages 52–3 and 90–1) instead of on your cat's body (or aura), using a pointer, with your non-dominant, non-dowsing hand, and asking one by one if each chakra needs balancing.

Once you discern a chakra that requires balancing, you may then send the appropriate coloured light (for example, red for the root chakra) to the chakra, and ask that it "Come into perfect balance, with any imbalanced energy to be released to be transmuted by the spiritual."

Please note that more than one chakra may require balancing, and I usually ask to be shown the "priority" chakra to be balanced to maximize the benefits of my healing sessions. As a beginner, though, feel free to balance the chakras as you receive them and not to get too caught up in the rest unless you already understand it.

Your Cat's Food and Water

You can create a positive spin over your cat's food and water, and this can be done for yourself as well. To begin, dowse over your cat's food and ask to be shown the "spin" of the food. If it is not organic, the chances are it will have a negative spin, and it could still have a negative spin even if organic.

If this is the case, then take your pendulum and force a spin to the right while you hold it over the food, and ask the dowsing system to change the spin of your cat's food to a positive one. Then, when you feel you have done it long enough, stop and re-ask for the spin of the food. If you've done it long enough, it should now be spinning positively.

You can do this with any type of food, drinking water, treats, supplements or medications your cat consumes. Any items should hold the positive spin once you have changed them to a positive one – unless some type of non-beneficial energy (geopathic, electromagnetic, microwave or thought form) has affected them after they have been changed.

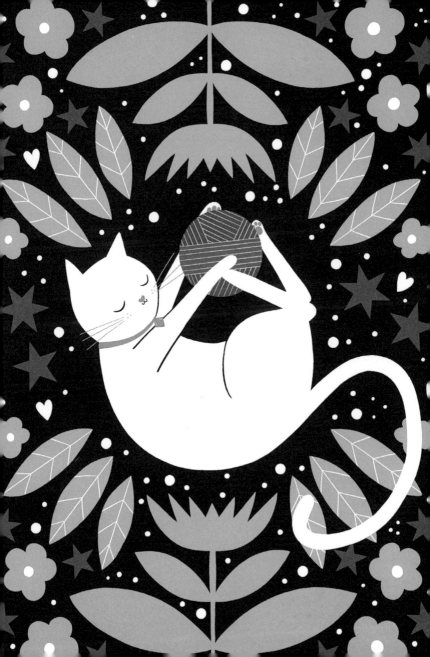

CONCLUSION

It is my hope that the techniques and information within this book will help you when working with your cat for healing and wellbeing. While this book is by no means exhaustive, it should give you and your cat a foundation to work with on your (and her) healing journey. I wish you the best as you proceed, and I always love to hear feedback from my readers and students, so please feel free to share on my website or social media. On the following pages, you will find additional information and resources should you wish to further your study. Enjoy the new and/or deeper connection you have with your feline companion!

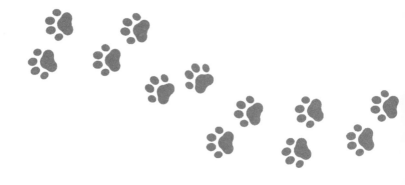

ABOUT THE CONTRIBUTORS

Lynn McKenzie is an expert in the animal intuitive and energy healing fields with over 30 years of experience. Through her signature Animal Energy® Certification Training programme in Sedona, Arizona, Lynn has built a global reputation, helping others identify, foster and embody their inherent gifts. She also offers programmes on spiritual growth, personal transformation, psychic development, clairvoyance mastery and chakra healing (see overleaf). She is also the author of *Bark, Neigh, Meow: Awaken to the Transformative Wisdom of Your Companion Animal to Activate Your Soul's Highest Calling.* Visit her at LynnMcKenzie.com.

Sian Summerhayes is an artist and illustrator currently living and working in the Cotswolds, UK. Inspired by her local countryside and homely cottage life in rural England, Sian's illustrations are charming, colourful and decorative. Depictions of wild flowers, quirky trees and meandering foliage create pretty landscapes and cosy cottage scenes. Dogs, cats, animals and birds feature heavily throughout her illustrations and have become a trademark of her work and pattern-led style. Sian also sells prints and cards of her illustrations as well as a selection of homewares. Visit her at siansummerhayes.com.

RESOURCES FOR READERS

Now that you are equipped with this information, you may want to go deeper on your healing journey with your cat and expand your knowledge even further.

There are two free resources that will help you open to deeper healing and connection with your feline companions as well as with every aspect of your life.

1. Making the Heart Connection with Your Animal Companions
This training course will help you open even further to deeper connections with your cats as well as with every aspect of your life. It's a six-part audio series with a workbook and webinar.
https://lynnmckenzie.com/training/

2. How to Master Animal Communication
This is a 90-minute webinar that covers: the three paths to animal communication mastery and how to know which is the best and easiest path for you; the number-one skill you must master to expand your animal communication and feel 100 per cent confident in your abilities; the key ingredient to confidently understanding your animal companions so you always know what they truly want; and the animal communication energy secret that is often missed but instantly makes you feel closer to your animal companions.
www.AnimalEnergyCertification.com

Lynn McKenzie offers in-depth training programmes and home study courses on a variety of topics to help you in the areas of healing, animal communication, psychic development and clairvoyance mastery, which you can learn more about on the website, LynnMcKenzie.com. If you feel called to deepen your connection and explore a new path and calling, take a look here.

BIBLIOGRAPHY

Books

Ted Andrews, *The Animal-wise Tarot*, Dragonhawk Publishing, 1999.

Margrit Coates, *Healing for Horses*, Rider, 2001.

Helen Graham and Gregory Vlamis, *Bach Flower Remedies for Animals*, Findhorn Press, 1999.

Lynn McKenzie, *Bark, Neigh Meow; Awaken to the Transformative Wisdom of Your Companion Animal to Activate Your Soul's Highest Calling*, Llewellyn Publications, 2021.

Martin J. Scott and Gael Mariani, *Crystal Healing for Animals*, Findhorn Press, 2002.

Diane Stein, *Natural Healing for Dogs and Cats*, Crossing Press, 1993.

Diane Stein, *The Natural Remedy Book for Dogs and Cats*, Crossing Press, 1994.

Online Sources and Websites

Daisy Foss, '7 Angels to Call Upon for Your Chakras', *Soul & Spirit*
www.soulandspiritmagazine.com/7-angels-call-upon-chakras/

Lynn McKenzie, Crystal Healing for Animals Home Study Program
www.lynnmckenzie.com/crystal-healing-for-animals/

Lynn McKenzie, Healing and Understanding Your Animal Companions through the Chakras™
Home Study Program
www.lynnmckenzie.com/healing-through-chakras/

Lynn McKenzie, The Chakra Balancing Method™ Home Study Program
www.lynnmckenzie.com/cbm/

Lynn McKenzie, *Animal Wellness* magazine author page
https://animalwellnessmagazine.com/author/lmckenzie/

Lynn McKenzie, *Equine Wellness* magazine author page
https://equinewellnessmagazine.com/author/lmckenzie/

Kathleen Prasad website
www.AnimalReikiSource.com

Penelope Smith website
www.AnimalTalk.net

INDEX

AUTHOR ACKNOWLEDGEMENTS

Thank you to all of my teachers, human and animal, with love and gratitude; especially to my beloved golden retriever, Jiggs, who came to me in the early 1990s to teach me, guide me and transform me. I had no idea what was in store for my life, and without your arrival I'd still be in a "normal" career and my current (and growing) body of work would not exist.

PICTURE CREDITS

All illustrations by Sian Summerhayes, © Welbeck Publishing Group: pages 6, 8, 21, 29, 48, 52–3, 76, 84, 90–1, 97, 102, 120, 125, 135.

ShutterstockPhotoInc: Ala Sharahlazava 31; Alena Solonshchikova 57, 61, 65, 69, 73, 81, 85, 89, 108, 117, 119, 123, 129; Anne Mathiasz 54–88; Arvila 35, 64, 88, 109; Chipmunk131 19; CloudyStock 12, 17, 44, 45, 93, 94, 95, 96, 98, 99, 100, 101, 102, 103, 104, 118; Dervish45 18, 19, 24, 68, 72, 80; dobrypies 25; Hein Nouwens 51; J.FLA 122; jelisua88 4–5, 92–6, 98–105; Kubko 46; Mark Rademaker 136; Mary Erskine 1, 131; Omeris (pawprints throughout); PonaOlga 5; Zanna Art (cat numerals throughout); Zuieva Oleksandra 25.

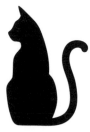